Choosing Wellness

Unconventional Wisdom for the Overwhelmed, the Discouraged, the Addicted, the Fearful, or the Stuck

Eileen T. O'Grady PhD, RN, NP

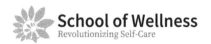

School of Wellness
Revolutionizing Self-Care

Publisher's Cataloging-In-Publication Data
(Prepared by The Donohue Group, Inc.)

Names: O'Grady, Eileen T., 1963- author.
Title: Choosing wellness : unconventional wisdom for the overwhelmed, the discouraged, the addicted, the fearful, or the stuck / Eileen T. O'Grady, PhD, RN, NP.
Description: [McLean, Virginia] : School of Wellness, [2021]
Identifiers: ISBN 9781736107409 (trade paperback) | ISBN 9781736107416 (ePub)
Subjects: LCSH: Self-care, Health. | O'Grady, Eileen T., 1963---Health. | Well-being. | Mind and body. | Alternative medicine.
Classification: LCC RA776.95 .O47 2021 (print) | LCC RA776.95 (ebook) | DDC 613--dc23

Library of Congress Control Number: 2021902532

Cover by Danijela Mijailovic

Printed in the United States of America

This book is dedicated to every person I have ever encountered who has met and overcome adversity or set out on the arduous journey to intentionally alter their life's direction and daily experience. Their stories, honesty, strength, and resilience have not only carried and expanded me; they have provided the jet fuel to write this book—and I thank each and every one of them.

ACKNOWLEDGEMENTS

Humayun Zeya, my husband and love who has always unconditionally supported me on my uncertain quests. My sons: Liam Zeya, whose astonishing maturity helped me to see that coaching techniques work on teenagers. Thank you for listening to me and giving me your thoughtful opinion on wellness topics and remedies for self-defeating behaviors, as well as for persuading me to commit to Google calendar!

Thanks also for the four single-spaced pages of feedback on my public-speaking skills. And Conor Zeya, who listened to my stories and how I see the world and always offered up a more chill, more accepting, and less judge-y approach. Your unwavering honesty and ever-present positive attitude, encouragement, and innocence greatly enhances my life. Your tech wizardry is inspiring.

Profound thanks to my huge-hearted friends and family—you know who you are, but I am listing anyway!

Everyone from Top of the Park, Fiona Druy, Kate Early, Jean Johnson, Maria Barnett, Lynn Brallier, John Cardona, Lin and Carly Amar, Pam Culvahouse, Kevin and John O'Grady, the entire Phoenixville O'Grady Clan, Sherra and Bob Mills, Loretta Ford, Dawn Adams, Janet Brightly, Becky and Liz Brumfield, Janet and Renee Thomas, Anne Blouin, Carolyn Buppert, Kathy Rowe, Marybeth Ryan, Ellen Politi, Anne Turner, Maigraid Lean, Nancy Rudner, Sally Strackbein, Tom Boland, Gwen Kinsey, Deb Gardener, Vernice Jones.

The folks at National Nurse Practitioner Symposium Mark Stone and Ann Clay, Chris Simpkins, Karin Walser , NPACE, Judy Collins, Polly Bednash, Nancy Sharp, Sparrow Hart, Anne Durand, Kate Malliarakis, Robbie White, Lydia Ketkar, Heather Glick, Amy Dobson, Julie Fowler, Carol Vernon, Paul Tschudi, Dorothy Schilder, Carolyn Stewart, Cathy McCarthy, Micheline Tusenuis, Victoria Esposito, John Greer, Helena Healy, Katie Hanusik, Char Shallow, Joanne Singleton, Balbina and Felix Soto, and Louise Young.

AUTHOR'S NOTE

I spent six years writing this book in fits and starts. I struggled mightily with the voice, as I in no way have the answers or rules that apply to the wild diversity of experiences in this messy world we live in. These are the hard-fought lessons I learned: a bumpy, imperfect journey that is my own. My sincerest wish is that you, who may be struggling, dissatisfied, or stuck in self-defeating behavior, will discover in reading this book a more direct path for yourself in achieving high-level wellness. I write as honestly and vulnerably as I can in the hopes that you find a ladder out. My qualifications are my knowing as a nurse practitioner, and more importantly, my brokenness. I push hard on the pursuit of wellness because I believe it's a damn important part of creating a beautiful life.

FOREWARD

Eileen has fully captured the idea that we all have more agency over our health than we realize or exercise. Her eloquence in these stories captures the central idea that we all must take ownership of our health and our lifestyles, as difficult as that is. Life is a journey, and this book leads one into the private spaces of a life, using short stories with all the milestones, pitfalls, and events that led to her behavioral changes, remarkable insights, and thoughtful analysis. It has many artfully crafted lessons of emotional intelligence and the introspection that is applicable to every life. It causes one to look into the mirror and honestly assess one's life, past, present, and future. Through these stories, Dr. O'Grady provides an important roadmap for finding one's way to high level wellness.

Humanity is front and center in every story. There is no escape, but to move… forward and ever more humanely, openly, and confidently. A must-read for anyone experiencing toxic levels of stress, burnout or overwhelm.

I hope this book catalyzes a self-care revolution.

Dr. Loretta Ford

Cofounder of the world's first nurse practitioner program
(1965, with Dr. Henry Silver at the University of Colorado)

Contents

1 CHOOSING WELLNESS

The nurse who took care of my sixteen-year-old brother John changed my life. I was only eleven when he was hospitalized for ileitis, and I was scared that the one person in my family I could count on was dying. He had been in Columbia Hospital in New York City for months and had lost a lot of weight, but no one would tell me why.

That was typical for my family. I would not have believed my parents even if they had tried to explain.

I was feeling small at the foot of his bed in the overcrowded hospital room when a young nurse walked in. I have never forgotten her kind voice when she asked if anyone had any questions, or the calm competence she exuded as she confidently calibrated the machine inflating the other patient's collapsed lung. I could see she knew the truth about my brother, his roommate, and all the other patients up and down the hallway.

Choosing Wellness

I wanted to know what she knew, and I suddenly saw my future—just as if I had been picked up by a hawk and delivered to my destiny. The commitment, the vow, the college major—my life's direction was all decided in that single moment.

I would know what she knew. I would be that nurse. I would radiate that same calm competence. I just did not realize the incredible journey it would take to get me there.

Within months, I was a candy-striper, a hospital volunteer who visited patients and assisted the staff. I never doubted my calling; never questioned my core identity as "nurse." It has been the lens through which I see the world.

John did not die during that hospitalization. Even though his symptoms continued, he eventually came home. But he never fully recovered until two years later, when he hitchhiked 3,000 miles away from our troubled home and his five younger siblings, for whom he felt responsible. His escape was his cure.

I did not escape until I, too, was eighteen and left for nursing school, where I eventually collected degrees and worked as a nurse practitioner for decades. Unlike John, though, my escape did not cure my lifestyle-generated maladies. I had to do that intentionally over the course of my adult life.

Nevertheless, my nursing career was exciting and extensive. I taught orthopedics to Peace Corp medical officers all over the world, I worked in rural Peru during a cholera epidemic. I served as a hospital nurse, a summer camp nurse, and worked at homeless shelters and academic health centers. I taught the next generation of nurse practitioners.

Somewhere along the way, I realized what I was doing no longer felt impactful enough. Where a clinical setting had once made me feel alive, it now left me drained, restless, and unhappy. Nursing had lost its meaning and purpose for me—and I did not know why.

I had studied adult-development theory, so I knew my feelings of being unanchored or dissatisfied might indicate a growth spurt. Maybe my way of living had become too small; maybe I needed a new challenge—not necessarily a new profession but a new mindset about my approach to life. A molting.

I asked myself: What about my current job feels constricting? "Writing prescriptions" popped into my head. Something about that part of my job felt deeply unsatisfying. Where do I want to grow? What do I want to do more/less of? With my unique education and experiences, how can I be most impactful?

The more I reflected, the more I realized I did not want to keep working in the traditional American medical model. We need that system; it is important but insufficient. I wanted something more.

Do I need a long vacation or a new vocation? I did not know how to answer that question.

Choosing Wellness

I wanted to fix the relationship I had with myself. I was drawn to the idea of a vision quest, undertaken by young Native American men entering adulthood.

I was not young, male, or on the verge of entering adulthood, but I certainly wanted to discover new meaning and purpose to my life. I found a guide who organized vision quests in the New Mexico wilderness.

My husband begged me not to go. "Four days and nights in the deep forest without food or shelter? I am begging you—go anywhere else. How about an ashram in India?"

But I simply had to do it, so I said good-bye to my small children and husband and flew to New Mexico. I felt some trepidation during the flight as I thought about what was ahead. I felt conflicted and selfish for leaving my family. I questioned myself, "who does this?" The pull to be alone was magnetic and overrode all the angst. I had been living a life with no white space for decades, every minute filled with course work, rescuing relatives, and building my career. What would it be like to spend four days with myself without numbing agents, busy-ness, or distractions?

Most people, I learned, went into the experience afraid of sleeping alone in the forest with no food or no protection from scorpions, snakes, or other creatures.

I was afraid of coming face-to-face with what I had been running from my whole life: being alone with myself.

I headed into the wilderness equipped only with a sleeping bag and a backpack filled with a jacket, tarp, notebook, pen, water vessel, and flashlight. I had no music, reading material, or anything else to distract the mind. I would only experience solitude fully for the first time in my life.

Two days in, I felt a little shaky from lack of food. I thought of all the important people in my life, one by one. I had a one-sided conversation with each of them as if this was the last conversation I would ever have with them.

When I started with my husband and sons, fierce, strong love poured out. I had feelings I had not even realized I felt before. I knew I loved my family, of course, but I had never contemplated the magnitude of their importance in my life, or how incredibly beautiful it was to acknowledge the deep, mutual affection that bound us all together.

Continuing, I "talked" to each one of my five siblings. Then I came to my mother, who had passed away a little over a year earlier. I expected to feel some version of sadness. Instead, I ripped into her. I called her names, sobbing and shaking with fury. My rage was like a tape worm—I kept pulling it out, but it seemed to have no end. I just kept going until nothing was left in me.

All that intense fury surprised and frightened me—I had not even known I was angry! I felt raw, yet wonderfully cleansed, as if someone had scrubbed my insides with a wire brush.

That experience did more for my wellbeing than any combination of medical treatments ever had or could. For the first time, I felt healed. And that healing crystalized why I had gotten so dissatisfied with my work. I spent most of my time writing prescriptions and telling people what to do, but it was not working. Not for them or me.

In my nurse-practitioner education, I learned to look at the whole person in their wider environment. But in my actual practice, I doled out advice in seven-minute visits that made no sense, given my patients' living situations. Inner-city Washington DC could be a toxic environment: street crime, nothing but fast-food restaurants, and inadequate transportation. Advising someone who lived there to pursue a healthy lifestyle teetered on magical thinking.

Rather than match symptoms and diseases to a pharmacologic remedy, I wanted to understand people's life experiences so I could guide them to become as whole as possible within their circumstances.

That insight gave me clarity. I wanted to practice nursing in a way that integrated everything I knew. I wanted to help adults change so I could transition them off prescriptions rather than write them.

The vision quest worked, but not in the way I expected. I came out of that wilderness with a deep self-knowledge. I could be still. I could be alone with myself. I could even like my own company.

If I could brave hunger, nature, and aloneness, I could find the courage to create a nurse practitioner/coaching practice that combined evidence-based healthcare and holistic healing.

I could draw on both my conventional and unconventional wisdom. I could emphasize the power of individual choice and the need for outside support.

I could choose wellness—and I could help other people do the same.

2 THE METAL SOUP LADLE AND EMOTIONAL REGULATION

I was a grown woman with multiple degrees and a family of my own when I undertook the vision quest. By then, it had been decades since my mother's metal soup ladle made me run away and hide in my bedroom closet, eyes closed tight, heart pounding, the taste of bile in my mouth. The dark may have frightened me, but not as much as my drunk, raging mother.

I knew she would hunt me down and beat me with that spoon.

My mother was an out-of-control maniac when she drank. We never knew what triggered her monthly episodes, or who would be the next target. They were frighteningly arbitrary. She would blow up at me or one of my five siblings over random slights. Even if I escaped her anger, it was just as awful hearing my brothers or sisters endure her rampage, which usually continued until she passed out—or my father piled us into the car and found a hotel for the night.

I was about nine the night she hit me with the ladle hard enough to give me a deep gash. My head would not stop bleeding. I needed sutures.

"Tell them that a neighborhood kid hit you with a rock," my mother commanded as my father and I left for the ER.

I did as I was told, understanding from that moment on that I was not to talk about what happened in my family. My mother was always remorseful and extremely kind to us all the next morning, as if the unspoken events of the prior evening had actually never happened.

That and other traumatic experiences made me feel completely powerless—I had no place to go and no one to tell.

All I could do to cope with my fear was shut down.

Nurse-Practitioner Coursework

Nurse practitioner education in the 1980s included taking classes with second year medical students. I had little preparation for this kind of academic rigor and had never taken bio or organic chemistry, so when the work mounted, I felt in-over-my-head. I shut down, became quiet and distant. My classmates learned to leave me alone when instead of my usual warm and friendly self, I met them with a cold, sealed-off version of me. I never explained the ice out—I did not understand it myself—so, not surprisingly, I developed a reputation for being moody.

That moodiness sabotaged my relationships and stunted my growth in profound ways. My unpredictable responses—charming one minute, aloof the next—made me wholly unsafe to interact with. I recall responding like a cold fish to a friend's funny story, whose mother, I later learned, was terminally ill at the time. She had not mentioned it because she did not know how I would respond.

Looking back, I cannot blame her. I was unaware of my own emotions at the time, let alone the effect they had on others, and I had no idea how my childhood trauma influenced my adult behavior. My low emotional intelligence and erratic behavior made it impossible for anyone to give me the compassion and connection I so desperately needed.

It was not until years later that I unraveled my moodiness. My childhood's cycle of violence and silence had taught me to stuff down my own feelings, and I had continued that behavior in my adult relationships. This is how feelings work when they go unacknowledged, unexpressed and unmetabolized. They burrow. They grow. They come out sideways. Pushing intense emotions underground served me beautifully as a child but was devastating my adult life.

Once I had to learned to see this pattern, I could deactivate my dysfunctional emotional autopilot. As soon

The Metal Soup Ladle and Emotional Regulation

as I notice fear rising, I now ask: "What am I afraid of?" and then consider what steps will help me dispel it: talk to a good listener, get quiet in nature, or just give myself permission to fail at something new. Learning to take full responsibility for my emotional landscape was my first step into self-empowerment.

Thankfully, I've consciously reshaped old, reactive habits into new growth patterns. Metal soup ladles no longer send me running for the closet. I now reach out for help rather than retreat when I am stressed or afraid. And people can trust I will communicate with them no matter the circumstances.

The more aware I became, the closer I grew toward becoming who I wanted to be: someone surrounded by love, trust, and strong connections in all aspects of my life.

When our own behavior is no longer serving us, we can hunt down its origins and choose to change and grow.

3 WHEN HELP ISN'T HELPFUL

I spent my entire life trying to help my older sister Ellen, who had been drinking since she was thirteen. It got so serious my parents admitted her to an inpatient treatment center when she was seventeen.

I was alarmed by the psychiatric ward's heavy metal doors that prevented the zombie-like residents from getting out. But Ellen had not been subdued into zombiehood by tranquilizing drugs, so she cried nonstop and begged to go home when I visited.

Since I looked up to her as my "cool" big sister, and had my heart set on a career in nursing for three years by then, I felt it was my job to bring her comfort, alleviate her pain, fix her life, and clean up her constant mess. So when, a week into rehab, Ellen asked me to bring her a note from her friend "Joe," who couldn't visit, I said, "Sure." As soon as I saw the envelope, I knew it contained drugs.

When Help Isn't Helpful

But I was only fourteen, and in my untrained, loving-sister mindset, I felt compelled to do something—anything—to help Ellen in that locked ward.

"At least they'll take the edge off that miserable place and give her some comfort," I told myself, bringing her the envelope.

The treatment center kicked her out the next day. She had taken everything in the envelope all at once. Neither consequence had ever occurred to me; I mean, why would anyone get so obviously high that everyone would notice?

I had no idea what addiction was.

Ellen was relieved, but my parents were enraged. I was stunned and ashamed. I had only wanted to help. I did not know I had actually enabled her death wish, or that her self-destructive drive was like a train plowing down the tracks, obliterating everything in its path.

I never told anyone what I did.

My "helping" instinct runs deep, but at that time I had no knowledge or tools to do anything but act on my pity. Would her life have turned out differently if I had reined it in? I never did, even though the havoc Ellen unleashed often frightened me. It seemed like everything she touched got broken, diminished, or went missing: my prescription glasses, my shoes, my favorite sweater. Or the time she drove away in the family car and returned home on foot.

No one ever saw the car again.

Choosing Wellness

When she dropped out of high school, my parents sent her to live with my oldest brother John, who had moved (hitchhiked from our home in New Jersey) to California. He was only twenty, and he convinced our parents that Ellen's alcoholism would improve if she moved. But she did not stay long. As we now know about addictions, this "geographic cure" failed, and she had soon run away from John to take up with a biker group at the age of seventeen.

I had no contact with her while she lived in California. I learned decades later that she had a baby boy who she gave up for adoption. She eventually moved back to New Jersey and earned her Licensed Practical Nurse (LPN) credential—which she lost when someone discovered she was stealing narcotics.

By then, I was twenty-one, working my first job as a Registered Nurse (RN) and housesitting on Capitol Hill in Washington D.C. for my employer's friend. Ellen asked if she could visit me.

I said yes, of course. How could I not? She was my sister. I did not know I had another choice. "Besides," I rationalized, "maybe if she sees me working and living on my own, it'll show her what stability looks like, and she'll become a normal person." Yes, I still believed in magic at that point. But not after coming home the first night to find strangers in the house, high on who knows what. Strangers—not just to me, but to Ellen. She had met them wherever she had gone to buy drugs.

When Help Isn't Helpful

I was terrified. The beautiful home I had been entrusted with was now filled with drug addicts. What had they already stolen? Were they leaving needles lying about? Would they hurt Ellen; would they hurt me? How could I get them out without causing any more harm?

I lied. "The owners are on their way home right now," I declared. "You all have to get out of here!"

They left peacefully enough, but my mind would not quiet down. I had tried to help my sister once again, and it had, once again, backfired spectacularly.

When would I learn?

Apparently, not soon. Again and again, I tried everything I could to fix her, to show her the way, to prop her up, to finance her—anything to make her be someone else, someone she wasn't, someone who didn't continually threaten to ruin her life, or mine. But no matter what I did—with love, humor, pleading, generosity—it was never enough.

It never could be.

Ellen eventually contracted AIDS. She had a second child, but when the boy was abused by her drug-addicted boyfriend, the courts stepped in.

Testifying at her hearing was excruciating; I had to choose between betraying my sister, whom I had pledged to help at all costs, or her two-year-old son, my adorable nephew. Ellen actually made it easier for me by disappearing for days at a time and leaving the boy in one unsafe situation after another. In the end, despite her pleading and promises, I knew down to my bones that she could never take care of her child anymore than she could take care of herself.

I testified against her. The state awarded custody to the paternal uncle and aunt (my nephew's father's sister). Ellen never even showed up for the hearing.

I was drowning in shame, stress, and pain. Ellen's disregard for her own safety exhausted and infuriated me, but I could not stop myself from trying, trying, trying to "fix" her. "This is my world," I reasoned. "These are the cards I was dealt. This is just... life."

Five years after Ellen brought those drug addicts into the D.C house, I found Lynn, my skilled, loving therapist. She only had to listen to me vent about the hot mess I called my sister for a few minutes before she began prodding me toward a profound realization: taking responsibility for other people without having authority over their actions is a lose-lose situation.

I had taken responsibility for repairing Ellen's bad decisions and felt compelled to make her well. Yet I had no authority, no agency, no control whatsoever over her actions, her emotions, or her inner demons. I could not change Ellen's life—only she could do that. I had to put down that burden and let her be who she was. I had to accept that the only things I could change were me and my life.

It was that simple.

When Help Isn't Helpful

With Lynn's help, I planned how to tell Ellen, for the first time, the way I truly felt. "Share your full truth from a place of love and radical acceptance," she advised. "But expect tears."

I invited my sister to my apartment in Arlington, Virginia. We sat together on my gray Ikea couch. I faced her, took a deep breath, and dove in.

"I love you, Ellen, I love you very much. And I'm sorry for all the chaos and trauma you've experienced in your life.

"I'm sorry addictions have consumed you and destroyed everything you hold dear. I hate that you have AIDS. I'll never stop hoping for a cure, but I understand your decision not to seek treatment. I do. I really do.

"I know how mightily you've suffered, and I know you felt betrayed when I testified against you. As hard as it was for me to do, I know it was harder for you to lose your parental rights and your child.

"But even that can't compare to the pain you must feel now, knowing you have to say goodbye forever to your beautiful little boy."

By then, we were both weeping. And we let the silence say what we couldn't voice aloud: her son had contracted HIV, and though he was reasonably healthy at the time, the disease was a death sentence in the 1980s and '90s.

"I promise I'll look after him and love him," I said when I could talk again. "I promise he won't suffer… and he won't die alone."

"Thank you!" she cried, grabbing me in a powerful hug.

That was my first experience with radical acceptance. I completely surrendered to the facts of Ellen's life.

As gut-wrenching as it was, I let Ellen know she was loved, not judged. I accepted her mental frailty, her physical brokenness, her unmoored morality. That was just who she was.

She was relieved by my acceptance. I was relieved by my freedom.

In that moment—in the instant I abandoned my misplaced responsibility to fix her—my rage dissipated. The liberation was palpable.

I was finally free. I had a choice.

4 FROM CIGARETTES TO RUNNING SHOES

When I started smoking cigarettes at age twelve, it had been more by default than by choice. Everyone in my family smoked. By age nineteen, I was up to a pack a day. Quitting never crossed my mind, until I took up running. Those two habits—the one I had developed over seven years, and the one I had never considered before—obviously conflicted.

We are all creatures of habit; we have to be. Habits make life easier. They do not require conscious effort or cognitive load, so they free up our attention for other things. I do not think about brushing my teeth every day—I just do it.

When I arrived at college, I did not exercise regularly. In fact, I had never played sports or had any interest in movement at all.

When my fun-loving lab partner Mike found out, he was shocked. "How could anybody not take care of their body?"

Choosing Wellness

A fitness buff, Mike was bewildered by my languid lifestyle and tried to convert me, constantly lecturing me about how working out increased energy, diminished pain perception, relieved stress, improved sleep. He went on and on and on.

At first, I resisted exercise because it seemed so unfamiliar. My family never had any concern for nutrition or health. School lunches were cream cheese and jelly on Wonder Bread with potato chips on the side. We snacked on junk food. My parents never walked anywhere, let alone went to a gym or exercise class. They led completely sedentary lives.

Even before I left for college, I knew I did not want to be like that; I just was not sure what I needed to change to avoid their path.

When I finally escaped to the real world, I was astonished at how many other people focused on good health. My peers not only exercised, they ate salads and yogurt. I watched them with interest and started eating better, and with Mike's constant pushing over the course of a year, I decided exercise was something else worth trying.

Without telling anyone for fear I would flame out, I started to run. At first, I only ran a block. Then two. A few blocks eventually stretched into a mile.

By then I thought of myself as a runner, so I replaced my cheap sneakers with real running shoes.

I was hooked.

From Cigarettes to Running Shoes

I loved the rhythm of my feet hitting the ground and how my leg muscles hardened. I discovered what people meant by "runner's high" and felt a thrill when I beat my distance goals. But as the distances increased, I got uncomfortably winded. My pack-a-day habit conflicted with my five-mile-a-day running habit.

That winter of my second year of college, I developed serious bronchitis. Just stepping out into the cold burned my lungs. My coughing fits made it impossible to run.

And yet, I still smoked.

Then one day, as I lit a cigarette in the frosty cold, I suddenly recognized the undeniable connection: every cigarette fed the bronchitis and robbed me of breath.

I had a decision to make: which was more important to me, smoking or running? I stamped out that cigarette and have not had another since.

Did I crave cigarettes after I quit? Yes I did. I would ask smokers to exhale their smoke and bad breath into my face and that quickly aborted the craving. It worked every time. Changing any habit, good or bad, is not a one-time decision. I had to re-decide every day as doubt crept in; I had to continually weigh the pain caused by the habit against the pain of changing it. It was a minute-by-minute recommitment to a compelling destination, to become a runner. Vague goals like "wanting to feel better" didn't have the emotional heft to drown out my critical inner voice nagging me to get off my exhausting new path.

Only a compelling and specific destination could sustain my effort: I wanted to run.

The Habit Cascade

Whether seeding a new habit or rooting out an old one, I have learned to laser-beam focus on one change at a time. When I started running, I made that the center of my attention. Years later, when I weaned myself off a six-pack-a-day soda habit, I did not attempt any other challenges. I knew willpower was a finite resource. If I drew on it too much, I would have set myself up for failure, like people who try to change their eating habits and start exercising at the same time. It is better to firmly establish one habit, then cultivate another.

This one running habit I picked up at age nineteen has stuck with me consistently over decades. It made me a daily exerciser because I am terrible at moderation—it is far easier for me to be all-in everyday than to manage an every-other-day habit. This important experience has had a profound impact on the quality of my life. Learning how to replace one habit with another reminds me I always have a choice. I can make a decision over and over and over again until I'm in cruise control.

5 WATCH FOR THORNS

When I was steeped in worry or anger over Ellen, I had not been my best self. Cortisol, the stress hormone, flowed through my organs. This put me into a constant fight-or-flight state, which is about as anti-choice as anyone can get. All that high anxiety sucked me dry and made me cranky, bitchy, and stressed-out—and justified, at least in my own mind, my nightly glass of wine, which often turned into an entire bottle.

I did not know it at the time, but I scored four-out-of-ten on the Adverse Childhood Event (ACE) scale, which meant I had experienced toxic-level physical and emotional trauma during my formative years. Adverse childhood events include neglect, physical or sexual abuse, and witnessing domestic violence or substance abuse.[1]

Adverse Childhood Events

During your first 18 years of life:[2]

1. Did a parent or other adult in the household often or very often:
Swear at you, insult you, put you down, or humiliate you?
or
Act in a way that made you afraid you might be physically hurt?
Yes No   If yes enter 1 _____

2. Did a parent or other adult in the household often or very often:
Push, grab, slap, or throw something at you?
or
Ever hit you so hard that you had marks or were injured?
Yes No   If yes enter 1 _____

3. Did an adult or person at least 5 years older than you ever...
Touch or fondle you or have you touch their body in a sexual way?
or
Attempt or actually have oral, anal, or vaginal intercourse with you?
Yes No   If yes enter 1 _____

4. Did you often or very often feel that:
No one in your family loved you or thought you were important or special?
or
Your family didn't look out for each other, feel close to each other, or support each other?
Yes No   If yes enter 1 _____

5. Did you often or very often feel that:
You didn't have enough to eat, had to wear dirty clothes, and had no one to protect you?
or
Your parents were too drunk or high to take care of you or take you to the doctor if you needed it?
Yes No   If yes enter 1 _____

6. Were your parents ever separated or divorced?
Yes No   If yes enter 1 _____

7. Was your mother or stepmother:
Often or very often pushed, grabbed, slapped, or had something thrown at her?
or
Ever repeatedly hit at least a few minutes or threatened with a gun or knife?
Yes No   If yes enter 1 _____

8. Did you live with anyone who was a problem drinker or alcoholic or who used street drugs?
Yes No   If yes enter 1 _____

9. Was a household member depressed or mentally ill, or did a household member attempt suicide?
Yes No   If yes enter 1 _____

10. Did a household member go to prison?
Yes No   If yes enter 1 _____

Add up your "Yes" answers: _____ This is your ACE score.

Watch for Thorns

Adverse child events and their relationship to adult health status and social problems was discovered by accident, the way penicillin was found to be growing in a petri dish and killing bacteria when Fleming returned from vacation. In the 1980s, physician Vincent Fellitti with Kaiser Health was noticing that over half of his patients were dropping out of an obesity program. What made him curious was that the dropouts were successful in losing weight at first, and then began gaining weight. So, he interviewed those who left and discovered that the majority of them had experienced childhood sexual abuse.

Digging more deeply, he learned that many had been unconsciously using obesity as a shield against unwanted sexual attention, or as a form of defense against physical attack.

Up until this discovery, obesity was conventionally viewed as the problem, not the unconscious solution to other, far more concealed, problems. The prevalence and severity of these problems was totally unexpected. Since this original discovery, solid scientific evidence has shown that toxic stress in formative years has profound effect on a range of health issues.

The physical abuse and terror I endured from my binge-drinking mother put me at risk for such preventable chronic problems as diabetes, heart disease, and obesity. I was also prone to depression, substance abuse, violence and/or being a victim of violence—and even suicide.

Choosing Wellness

My brother John's Crohn's Disease was 100 percent stress-induced; it began clearing up as soon as he moved 3,000 miles away from home. Ellen contracted HIV due to her reckless behavior. Another sister intentionally overdosed; she only survived because someone found her in time.

The more adverse events we experience as children—and younger siblings tend to witness more of them—the more dysfunctional our behavior as adults. Childhood coping mechanisms like people-pleasing, using substances or overeating to soothe ourselves, isolating, keeping everyone at arm's length, all become counterproductive or even harmful when we grow up. We think we are protecting ourselves, but others see us as infuriating, secretive, or self-indulgent. They have no way of knowing our actions and words are hiding our hurt—even when they behave similarly, for similar reasons.

Most of us have no idea why we act the way we do. Our negative behaviors and thought processes are like thorns in our paws.

The medieval fable 'Androcles and the Lion' has a profound moral lesson for modern life. A lion's roaring day and night terrorized the village. People lived in constant fear and stayed indoors. By chance, Androcles the Shepard was up in the mountains one day herding his flock, when he heard whimpering coming from a cave. When he peered inside, there was the lion, lying on its side.

Watch for Thorns

Putting aside his fears, Androcles crawled into the den and carefully removed the thorn he found in the lion's paw.

The lion stopped roaring, and in gratitude became peaceful and shared his catch. Peace returned to the village. And Androcles made a friend for life. The primary law of nature is reciprocal kindness.

Like Androcles, I have learned to de-personalize bad behavior. The driver who cuts me off in traffic is not intentionally trying to harm me, so I do not let them feed my outrage or divert my attention from the road. Maybe their mother is in hospice. Maybe they suspect their spouse is cheating on them, or their child is fighting an addiction. Maybe they feel threatened by the young hire who wants their job.

Maybe their thorn comes from a four-or-higher Adverse Childhood Event score.

When I assume the other person has a thorn, I not only avoid compounding their pain, I keep my own stress levels down—which lets me be of help, if possible.

Everyone wins.

Always Assume Positive Intent

Attributing only positive intent to difficult people has been a game changer for me. I no longer assume anyone's bad behavior is due to something I did or said. I realize their words or actions are likely a manifestation of their own unaddressed, invisible source, which makes my stress and reactivity drop exponentially. Every time I "refuse the bait" I become as emancipated as the moment I discarded my need to "fix" my sister Ellen. I no longer stress myself out over things I cannot control or compound the other person's distress.

This mind-hack does not sweep conflict under the rug: it does not give me an excuse to go back to people-pleasing, accept someone's abusive or toxic words, or even ignore their bad behavior. It merely gives me a pause button so I can consider my most productive response.

When one of my graduate students did not turn in her paper, I did not question her work ethic or commitment to the class.

Assuming positive intent, I merely emailed her. "Is everything all right?"

She responded with a phone call. "I just gave birth prematurely!"

"I had no idea you were expecting! Congratulations!"

"I'll get the paper in as soon as possible," she promised.

"Don't push yourself," I advised her. "Take whatever time you need!"

Yet while I always start with kindness, I do have limits. When I noticed another student always had a different excuse for not turning in assignments, I called her on it. "If you want to stay in the class, you'll have to sign an agreement to accept an F if you don't meet the rest of the assignment deadlines."

Watch for Thorns

Many science majors have limited writing experience, so some just do not know how to succeed in graduate school. I always tried to meet them where they were and connect them with writing tutors, if necessary, but hold them accountable for their own progress. It was my way of acknowledging their thorn without enabling them or allowing their excuses.

Hurt lions are everywhere, roaring and rattling us with their pain. They may not have the wherewithal to choose how they act, but I do. By deciding to make kindness and compassion a habit rather than a special effort, I became able to skip anger's cortisol bath and ease the other person's pain, if only for a moment. And sometimes—not always, but sometimes—that raging beast transformed into a grateful person, or even a friend.

Wellness is always a choice.

Endnotes

1   Anyone can determine their Adverse Childhood Event Score (ACE) by taking the ten-question survey on-line. https://n.pr/3b9qKbZ

2   Adapted from: http://www.acestudy.org/files/ACE_Score_Calculator.pdf, 092406RA4CR

6 CREATE ROMANCE STANDARDS

Choosing wellness affects every part of who we are—even our love life. I once accepted a date with a man I had met at work, even though I had zero interest in him. I was still young, so it never occurred to me to say no to his dinner invitation.

The year was 1991, the place was Washington, D.C., and all anybody could talk about was Clarence Thomas' Supreme Court confirmation hearings and Anita Hill, who accused him of sexual harassment years earlier when they worked together.

"Brian" and I made small talk as we drove the fifty miles to dinner at a charming inn. After ordering, our conversation moved to who was telling the truth: Clarence Thomas or Anita Hill.

"I can't believe what a liar that woman is!" Brian said. "She shouldn't even be allowed to testify!"

Create Romance Standards

"Well," I responded, somewhat dumbfounded, "we can't know, can we? I'm a nurse, and I've had physicians try to grope and kiss me in hospital elevators. I didn't even know it was illegal. I'd never sent them any kind of interest signal; in fact, they were all exceedingly unattractive to me."

"It's so obvious she's lying," he said, as if I had not spoken. "She's just making things up with no evidence."

I suddenly realized I would rather be home on my couch alone, but I was fifty miles from my apartment, stuck with this creep for rest of the evening. I changed the subject but decided right then and there to never, ever accept an invitation from anyone again unless they were someone I would ask out myself.

In that moment, I made the wellness choice to take charge of my romantic life. No more waiting around for someone to notice me. If I wanted a date, I would ask for it.

When Brian pulled up to my apartment, he kissed my cheek and said he had had a great time. "I hope I can see you again, soon."

I could not get out of that car fast enough.

My new choice led me to ask myself better questions: Who do I want to date? What are my criteria?

Soon after, when "Sam" asked me to the movies, I was in a gray zone, unsure if I was interested in him. Then he said, "I'd like to take you to see Basic Instinct."

"Basic Instinct?!" I exclaimed. "Isn't that soft porn?! You want to take me to that on a first date? Thanks, but no."

So much for the gray zone. I felt empowered. I was Wonder Woman, zapping unqualified men with my wrist band.

Choice is good, I told myself.

Months later, I found myself interested in a tall, kind medical resident who rotated through my clinic once a week. We flirted a little. He left snacks on my desk. I was intrigued.

"Do you like modern dance?" he asked one day.

"I'm not sure, but I'll try it."

We saw the Harlem Dance Theatre, an edgy, enchanting production, at the Kennedy Center. Afterwards, we went to a landmark restaurant in a diverse and lively DC neighborhood I had never been to before. We stayed until closing, belly laughing as we shared our lives with each other. I recall thinking that although the Kennedy Center was not far from where Basic Instinct was playing, it was light years away.

I wanted to see the resident again, but a week went by, and then another without hearing from him.

Choosing not to wait, I called him.

"Hi," I said, trying to keep the trepidation out of my voice. "I haven't heard from you in a while. I'd like to take you to an Indian restaurant I've been wanting to try. Can I pick you up Saturday at seven?"

I did it! I asked a guy out for the first time in my life!

And he said yes.

Create Romance Standards

I picked him up. We had a beautiful time laughing and talking. Only later did I learn our Kennedy Center-and-dinner date had wiped out his resident's salary for the month. No wonder he had not called me.

Six weeks later, I polled my friends about how long it took them to know they loved somebody.

"Six to eight weeks," most of them said.

"If you're still trying to decide after a year, the answer is NO."

Nine months into the relationship, I arranged a picnic.

"I have stronger feelings for you than I've ever had for anybody," I admitted to my resident. "I think its time we stopped seeing other people. You know—be exclusive."

"Wait—" he said, straightening up and pulling back. "You're seeing other people? What in the world is this?!"

It was our first argument. He had assumed we were exclusive; I had assumed we needed to agree on that first.

Decades into our marriage, we are still trying to align our communication. I am so grateful that Brian provoked me to take full agency over who I would date!

7 FEED THE RIGHT WOLF

In Cherokee legend, an elder and his grandson were discussing why there is so much cruelty and violence in the world. The grandfather says, "I too, at times, have felt a great hatred for those who have taken so much with no sorrow for what they do. It's as if I have two wolves fighting inside me. So do you. One wolf is evil, angry, envious, sorrowful, regretful, greedy, arrogant, self-pitying, resentful, lying, pompous, superior, and egotistical. The other is joyful, peaceful, understanding, loving, kind, benevolent, gentle, empathetic, generous, honest, compassionate, faithful, and serene. It is hard to live with these two wolves inside me. They are constantly fighting to control my spirit."

The boy says to his grandfather, "How is it you never seem to get upset? Don't you ever feel angry?"

His grandfather replies, "Whenever something angers me, one of the wolves is full of fire, and wants to attack and act nasty. The other is calmer, thinks clearly, and makes better choices. But they're both always there."

And the boy asks, "But if they are always fighting, how do you know which wolf is going to win?"

"The one you choose to feed," his grandfather replies.

We all have two wolves fighting inside our heart. We cannot banish our negative wolf, but I have learned how to direct its power to serve my positive purposes.

I had spent four exhausting years jumping through fiery hoops to get a PhD I did not need—or even want by the time the end was in sight. As soon as I finished my dissertation, I could take my victory lap and move on.

But my PhD adviser kept moving the goalposts. She insisted on an extra analysis. It seemed like busy work to me, and the two other committee members, both well-regarded intellectual powerhouses, agreed it was unnecessary—but nevertheless mandatory. My resentment toward my advisor rose exponentially.

Fortunately, I had enough emotional awareness by that point to recognize I needed to do something about my bitterness; otherwise, I would just hamper my own ability to think clearly and work productively. I had to find a way over my emotional hurdle so I could vault my last academic one. I recalled reading that in the darkest moments of the Civil war, Abe Lincoln wrote—but never sent—insulting, vicious letters to his generals who kept making mistakes. After his death, aides discovered them in his desk.

I had found my solution.

When I opened my dissertation document every day, I headed directly to the acknowledgments page and wrote mean-spirited "tributes" about my adviser's punitive authority and general incompetence. Sometimes I just revised earlier comments; other times I wrote entirely new ones. Eventually, I had a whole page of nasty, irreverent, profane statements that captured everything I wanted to say to her but could not.

Once I had poured out my resentment, I turned to the real acknowledgements, the ones thanking the people I was most grateful for. I reread the beautiful tributes to my husband and classmates who helped me through the dissertation process. I lingered over my wishes for the son I was expecting. With my bitterness tamped down for the day, I filled myself with gratitude and anticipatory joy until, finally, I was ready to write. I finished my dissertation.

The day before my oral defense, I edited the acknowledgments page one last time. I trimmed all my nasty words to a single vanilla sentence that thanked my adviser for her time on the project. Period.

People do hurtful things, but I do not let their "slings and arrows" harm me. I choose instead to deflect their insults, avoid sending angry emails, and stop myself from being self-destructive or acting out. I have come to recognize that feeding my vicious wolf only provides temporary relief at best—and often complicates matters further.

Feed the Right Wolf

I alone am responsible for getting rid of resentments that corrode my body, relationships, and psyche. I started with the "Serenity Poem":

> Grant me the serenity to accept the
> things I cannot change,
> The courage to change the things I can,
> And the wisdom to know the difference.

But since the poem felt like an invitation to passivity, I created a more comfortable version for myself, putting the action steps in a more pragmatic sequence:

> Find the courage to change the things you can.
> Ask for the serenity to accept the things you cannot.

As part of that first step, I like to ask myself:

- Can I change what is going on?
- Can I find a remedy or a solution to the problem?
- Can I have a conversation with the person who is causing my distress?
- Do I need to be more open or shift my own attitude?

Those questions open up possibilities to move past conflict or improve—even a little bit—whatever is making me feel stuck.

Step two urges radical acceptance because sometimes I have control over a situation, but other times I do not. Acceptance is not approval; I need not like or agree with something to accept it. But embracing serenity empowers me to not be a victim—to choose an alternate emotional response and envision new ways to overcome obstacles.

Since I could not change the situation with my dissertation adviser, I needed to stop fighting it, let go of my resentment, get the work done, and put it behind me without guilt. It was not a once-and-done decision; I had to work at it every time I opened my dissertation document. But using the healthy trick I learned from Lincoln prevented more negative feelings from building up inside and spilling out in unpredictable ways. Maybe I was shouting into the void, but at least I gave voice to my feelings without hurting anyone.

Once out from under my adviser's thumb, I continued feeding the right wolf. I tried to imagine what motivated her to push me harder than necessary. Maybe she thought I had more ability than the average bear. Maybe she wanted me to see I could rise to a higher expectation. Whatever the real reason, assuming she had good intentions helped me release my animosity.

Believing otherwise would have fed the bad wolf.

My Favorite Mistake

Now that I have even more perspective on the ill-suited doctoral degree, I now refer to it as my favorite mistake. There is so much limitation that I alone created. I was not an engaged learner, I did not care and just wanted to get through it and skate by on the minimum. I had been in graduate school for so long, I would simply study the syllabus for each class, and only do what was getting graded! More crafty than smart, I learned to cut and paste the grading rubric and use it as the outline to write papers, ensuring I had all the requirements. I would write the same paper for each professor, changing the topics and a few references. I had moments of wonder during my dissertation, doing factor analysis and discovering interesting connections between variables. But these moments were so few, far apart, and short-lived. I was a student with the worst possible attitude, ensuring none of the faculty cared about me. I never attended graduation, and nobody from the program contacted me, asked me if I published my research, or needed mentoring. I did not allow anybody to invest in me as a person.

By the time the PhD diploma was mailed to me, it meant very little—and still does. The diploma is hidden away, and I've never wanted to be called "Dr. O'Grady." It was one of my last grand acts of approval-seeking, needing something outside of myself to let me know I was okay. My motives were inappropriate and I created this hostile climate for myself. It is my favorite mistake because, one, I am in awe of seeing what Brene Brown has done with her grounded research on shame and vulnerability. She used her dissertation to launch a lifelong career and made shame and vulnerability far-reaching and relevant to a wide swath of America. What could have happened If I had been engaged, respectful and studied a topic I cared deeply about—like self-care? And two, earning a PhD has opened so many doors for me. It demonstrates to others I have a legitimate claim to understanding research and the scientific process. It shows I have grit.

I first forgave myself; for putting myself through that, for being so disengaged, and for feeding the wrong wolf.

Then I forgave my adviser.

Forgiveness, Gratitude, Peace

I had occasion to put my new coping mechanisms to work when my husband and I renovated our house. What I thought would be a few months' inconvenience turned into an eight-month ordeal that included a fire, a flood, and the entire interior being painted a hideous color by mistake.

The electrician, named Sparky (honestly!), turned a light fixture on that I had covered with a towel and duct tape to keep it protected. While the ensuing fire was frightening, it caused minimal damage.

Weeks later, the painters had been painting the interior of the house for four days straight. I watched them work, nodding in approval. I was bewildered when they stared packing up their gear, as if they were leaving. Turns out, paint is ordered by number, not by name, and they had been given the wrong paint number. The entire interior of the house was painted bowling-alley-bathroom blue.

I saw them every day painting that hideous color and never said a word because I thought it was the primer. I imagine the painters over dinner with their families, their conversation about the crazy woman who watched them paint the entire house the wrong color and did not say anything!

Then, when they came back to repaint the entire inside of the house, an outdoor hose used to clean brushes was left on overnight. We were awoken in the middle of the night, in the basement, to the sound of cascading water pouring down the wall.

I was wholly unprepared for the disruption the project caused. We lived in two rooms, without a kitchen, with constant jackhammering, filth, and the opening of walls caused many large spiders to appear in the basement. My sons were five and seven, my husband and I both worked full time. I was so stressed I could not even laugh when my son's kindergarten teacher phoned, concerned about child abuse. He had told his class he lived in the basement and she was concerned, she wasn't sure if this was a referral to child protective services. I explained, through gritted teeth, that the whole family lived in the basement due to our ongoing, over-budget, botched renovation!

We were ecstatic with the results when the nightmare ended and we moved back upstairs into a beautiful new space, but I could not release my burning anger toward the contractor. I grew so furious every time I thought or talked about the renovation that the vein in my neck bulged, my nostrils flared, and I formulated mean-spirited revenge fantasies.

Choosing Wellness

After one particular rant, my husband said, "You need to forgive the contractor, so you can move forward."

After thinking that over for a few days, we invited the contractor's entire company over for lunch. Over a spread of baguettes and deli items, my family and I thanked each and every one of the company's twenty employees, including the back-office staff, who had never seen any part of the renovation.

"No one has ever done this before," the contractor told me. "On behalf of my staff and myself, thank you very much."

We parted on good terms without him ever knowing that this simple expression of gratitude was designed to help me get unstuck from my own psychic pain and distress—and it did. I have never again had a single negative thought or feeling about that contractor or the renovation.

Even better, the experience lowered my cortisol levels and blood pressure. I felt peaceful and calm as I cleaned up from the party; I had fed the right wolf, taken full responsibility for my inner reactions and emotions, and released the negativity affecting my wellbeing.

By choosing to forgive someone else, I healed myself.

It happens every time.

8 STOP THE BULLIES

I whole-heartedly believe kindness is the first defense when I have to deal with difficult people, but even kindness has its limits. When someone ignores the rules and boundaries, disregards the norms of civil behavior, does not care about fairness, or tramples on others to get what they want—we likely have bully behavior that must be dealt with swiftly. Confronting bullying behavior is hard, but it is the only way we can protect ourselves. Understanding how to handle difficult people keeps me from becoming paralyzed with fear in tense situations—like the one I faced as a hospital float nurse.

Float nurses are not deep clinical experts; they move around the hospital filling in where needed. One morning I had thirteen patients with a long list of procedures and medications to dispense. Somehow, I gave an insulin injection to a non-diabetic patient scheduled to go home.

Choosing Wellness

As soon as I realized my mistake (and it was a major screw up), I immediately told the nurses in charge. They were concerned for the patient, of course, but they were also worried about me. The attending physician had a reputation as a tyrant who often flew into rages—and he was on his way up to the floor at that very moment.

I did not know him, and I was sick at heart about potentially harming the patient and delaying her discharge. I was also stressed over my twelve other patients, who needed my attention.

The clock was ticking.

Yet first, I had to own my mistake to the physician, so when he arrived, his face in a furrowed scowl, I put my arm out forcefully and shook his hand.

"I'm Eileen O'Grady, the registered nurse who erroneously gave insulin to your patient scheduled to go home today. I've given her food and checked her blood sugar—it's eighty-five. I'm monitoring her symptoms closely and rechecking her blood sugar every hour.

"I'm so very sorry and so worried about this error. I'm also sorry for all the hassle this is causing you. Will you accept my apology, and do you agree with this remedy to keep her safe, or do you want to modify it?"

His brow relaxed, he said, "Yes, yes, yes, of course. I would like to know how this happened, but yes, that plan is sound. I think we'll keep her in the hospital until later this afternoon."

The floor nurses gasped. Even I was stunned at how fully owning my mistake and already being in-solution had shut down the physician's negative reaction or abusive behavior. Thankfully, having been trained to handle medical errors, I knew Marshall Rosenberg's Principles of Nonviolence: We are all compassionate by nature, need to belong, need recognition, and need to be free from fear. These four steps based on those principles can be used to effectively deal with difficult encounters:

1. **Give the facts** as if reporting the news. Avoid opinions, judging, or blaming. I had done that when I stuck out my hand and reported the situation.
2. **Describe feelings** using "I" statements. I had apologized and expressed regret without trying to avoid culpability.
3. **Express situational needs** in non-emotional terms. I had told the physician I needed him to approve or modify my treatment plan.
4. **Make your request**, but note that if steps one through three are not said before the "ask," your request can seem like a demand. That is why, even though it felt a bit redundant, I not only told him what I needed, I asked him to give it to me.

Most people jump right to number four, which disregards the needs and emotions of the other person. I took into consideration what the physician likely felt when he first learned about the mistake, and so immediately both shared his emotional concern for his patient and shouldered the responsibility with him. That empathetic gesture let me address his fear while immediately directing him to the solution. Had he resorted to hostile behavior, I was prepared to interrupt and shift his attention back to the patient and the solution.

Witnessing Bullies

Not long after earning my PhD, I was in a team meeting with about ten people: several physicians, a few other nurse practitioners, some nursing assistants, and our unit's receptionist. One of the physicians was criticizing one of the nursing assistants to the point that she froze—she clearly could not defend herself or even answer his accusations.

Looking around, I saw no one else would respond to his bullying, so I stood up, raised my hand palm out, and said, "This conversation stops right now. We don't name call on this team."

Then I turned to the nursing assistant. "Will you please step outside with me?"

Once in the corridor, I said, "You never have to endure behavior like that. Practice mental karate. Stop them midsentence and name their offensive behavior—just like I did."

"But I need this job! I can't just interrupt a superior like that. He's a physician! I don't have your position on the team. I wouldn't know how to do what you did."

"Yes, you do. We train other people how to treat us. I want you to teach the rest of the team to treat you with respect. It helps to have a few good lines at the ready. If you can't bring yourself to physically hold up your hand, you can always interrupt the bully in midsentence with a strong, 'Excuse me!'

"Excuse me! I have never let anyone speak to me like that, and I'm not going to start now.

"Excuse me! You need to step back. You are in my space.

"Excuse me! If you need to know right now, the answer is no.

"Excuse me! You need to stop. Belittling me will not help us find a solution.

"Excuse me! It feels like you're pressuring me into going your way."

Her eyes widened as I spoke. When I finished, she said, "Those are great ideas. I'm going to remember them."

By then we had moved to the break room, so I sat her down and gave her a few more tips for dealing with bullies:

- Only use "you" statements to keep the spotlight on what they need to change. This is a sharp departure from using "I" statements—with aggressive red line bully behaviors, deploy the "you".

- Do not engage—do not reason, argue, or offer explanations

- Redirect the conversation productively—OR declare it unacceptable and leave

That physician had clearly lost emotional control, unable to govern himself. He needed someone to stop him. Cutting him off mid-tirade and leaving gave him—and everyone else—time to calm down.

I sought him out in his office the next day. "What happened yesterday? We're trying to build a strong, healthy team. I'm wondering if I've overestimated you."

As he began to reiterate all his complaints about the nursing assistant, I stopped him again. "How does any of this help our team function any better? What good is a frightened team member?"

He blinked a few times and then grinned sheepishly. "You're right; I was a jerk. I'm sorry."

"Don't tell me. Tell her—at the next meeting. You humiliated her publicly; you have to apologize the same way."

He did.

Bullying comes in a thousand forms, but these common behaviors cross the line from rude to unacceptable when directed specifically at any one individual:

1. Yelling, cussing, or blaming
2. Name calling
3. Throwing things
4. Unwanted physical contact
5. Toxic gossip

Combatting bullies does not mean I have to dial back my humanity; rather, it challenges me to fully embrace it.

9 HOW TO SHUT DOWN OUR INNER CRITIC

Like everyone else, I have an inner critic who loves to remind me how incompetent I am. When I branch out and try new things, my deep skeptic sets up a slide show of memories from my personal Hall of Shame, narrated with comments like, "Who do you think you are?" and "What makes you think you can do that?" and "This will be another failure, just like trying out for the bowling team."

My father kept telling me I needed extracurricular activities on my transcript if I wanted to get into college. I did not play sports, sing in the chorus, or even work backstage on school productions. I spent most of my non-school time smoking weed—which does not really stimulate ambition. Then I remembered I had bowled a dozen or so times and was always scoring higher than others, so I decided to try out for the bowling team. Somehow, I convinced myself I would excel at it. How hard could it be?

Choosing Wellness

Arriving at the bowling alley, I had done nothing to prepare for the tryouts. The vibe was very tense, each of the students checking each other out. The coach (who was also my art teacher) was surprised I was there and was really rooting for me. After my first gutter ball, he approached me and told me to look at the center dot on the floor and aim for that. I did and got 8 pins down. Throughout the tryouts, he kept giving me tips—to flick my wrist, where to put my feet, and where to place my attention. I was doing okay, but nowhere near the other hard-driving serious bowlers at tryouts. In the end, the coach privately spoke to me about how much potential I had, and that if I worked hard, I could earn a spot on the team next year.

Despite the bowling coach's exceptional kindness, when I did not make the team, my inner critic immediately labeled me a loser. "Don't try out for things, you are a loser," she advised—then and forever more. "What if you fail? What if you get rejected? You know how much that hurts!"

I listened to that voice—of course, we all do to different degrees. I never tried out for anything again after my bowling tryout; in fact, I avoided all competition. Even when I started running, I felt secure knowing it was an individual activity. I never had to worry about failing, losing, or competing. That thinking continued to shape my choices for decades.

I did spin classes, high intensity cycling workouts on a stationary bike, because I did not have to compete against anyone else. But after seeing me nearly every day for four years, my spin instructor suggested I do the Seagull Century Ride, a pancake-flat, 100-mile ride along Maryland's eastern shore. Since it was a group ride, not a race, I decided to give it a try. I bought an expensive road bike, got a computer installed to track my mileage and time, and started doing longer and longer outdoor rides.

I set out on the day of the Seagull Century with shaky confidence about my ability to finish the course, but the excitement of 8,000 other riders in all kinds of costumes, angel wings, and tuxedos carried me through the miles. It seemed possible—even fun.

About two hours into the ride, the computer tracked my distance at eighteen miles. I did the math. At that rate, I would not be done for another ten hours—well after dark.

My inner critic unleashed a cruel and unchecked rant.

Who do you think you are?

Loser! You know you can't do this. You're too incompetent and weak.

You'll finish dead last. The staff will be annoyed; they'll be waiting for you so they can finish sweeping up.

The thoughts went on and on. I would never talk to another person the way I harangued myself that day, but I could not stop my inner critic. I let her continue her malicious monologue, bullying me, deriding me, trying to undermine me, even when she took it all the way back to high school and my bowling-team failure.

At that point in my life, I had no inner advocate to counter the criticism with my many achievements, or even offer positive affirmations such as, "Keep going! You can do this!" The chatter inside my head focused solely on my incompetence and how I was only 18 miles into a 100-mile ride.

I was blinking back tears when a woman pulled up beside me. "You're such a strong rider," she said. "I've been drafting you for ten miles. Can you believe we're almost halfway through?"

"What?! I thought we were at mile eighteen!"

"No, we're at mile forty-eight—only two miles from the halfway point."

"Wow, thank you! My bike computer is way off! Thanks for the kind words—and the mileage check!"

Nothing had changed, but I felt giddy, even elated. My self-talk instantly flipped from negative to positive, and my energy surged. I would finish in five hours as planned. I was not a loser; I actually *could* ride 100 miles in a day. I rode strong and exultant for the remaining fifty-two miles.

After the Seagull Century, I wondered, "How often have I let negative thoughts defeat me? How frequently did I rely on my own bad information? How many times had I let inner voices determine my reality?"

Since that day, I have worked to shut down my inner critic. Even though I know she is wrong, she still takes me by surprise and works hard to discourage me whenever I step out of my comfort zone. But I choose to disregard her more and more, and she no longer stops me from doing what I feel is right.

Manage Our Inner Critic

I once worked with a coach to build a presentation for a nonmedical audience. She suggested I practice with a group of neighbors and friends to gather feedback, so I invited a dozen people over for dinner before I gave them the talk in my living room.

As the day approached and my anxiety escalated, my inner critic kicked in with her usual tricks.

"Who do you think you are?" she carped. "Those people aren't interested in what you have to say."

The day arrived. Morning slipped into afternoon. The voice got louder and meaner. My body responded to the criticism as if it were something real, making me feel physically drained and vaguely ill. By three o'clock, I was so worked up by my self-generated shame storm I considered canceling the event.

But then I noticed what I was feeling, and realized it was just my inner critic, which, in my mind's ear, sounded like my deceased mother. I was criticized a lot by her as a child, and some of the phrases in my self-talk were very old and familiar. That gave me an idea.

I found a framed photograph of my mother. "You're not invited to my presentation," I told her, in a loving voice. I took the photo outside, placed it in the passenger seat of my car, and walked back into the house.

The voice disappeared.

My relief was instant and dramatic.

The evening was a complete success. My friends gave me valuable feedback on my presentation and let me know I had a great message to share. I have since delivered it to all kinds of organizations.

And I learned a valuable lesson: my body is an early warning system. As soon as I feel bile at the back of my throat, I need to immediately command my inner critic to shut up. When, despite my best efforts, my self-talk whispers, "Who do you think you are?" I tell it, "I'm a person who likes to challenge herself! I'm someone who likes to learn new things and stretch herself. I'm making you uncomfortable right now because we're in unfamiliar territory, but I can handle the challenge, so you're not welcome here. Just shut the *eff* up."

When I got in the car with my son the next day, he asked, "Mom, what's grandma's picture doing here?"

"She's helping me to work through some fear so I can be brave, and she is coming with us to soccer practice."

10 WHEN PEOPLE LET YOU DOWN

I met my friend "Donna" during my first years as a nurse practitioner on a three-week Peruvian medical mission to help cholera victims. We hit it off at the orientation and kept each other company during the four plane rides and treacherous, eight-hour drive up the Andes mountains. The tight bond we forged lasted a decade.

Living five states apart, we did not see each other often, but when we did, we always picked up right where we had left off, sharing candor and lots of belly laughs. I considered her such a dear friend I asked her to be one of my brides-maids. I invited her family for holidays, made sure she had plans for her first post-divorce Thanksgiving, and generally anticipated her needs.

Oddly, she rarely anticipated mine.

"Eileen, you're such a good friend to me," she used to say, "but I'm not one to you."

"Of course you are," I always replied.

One summer, Donna asked if she and her daughters could visit for a week in August. I was thrilled! I canceled my kids' camps, planned day trips, and arranged time off from work.

The day before they were supposed to arrive, Donna sent a text message: "Hey Eileen, we're not going to make it this year. The girls and I have been running all summer. We need some time to relax at home."

I stared at my phone in disbelief and disappointment, until finally, I was overwhelmed by a surge of anger. What kind of friend cancels an elaborately planned visit—by text message—on such short notice?

I was going to really tell her off when she called.

But she never did.

Donna and I have never had a live conversation since then. Our close relationship has devolved to her sending a "Happy Mother's Day" text every year, and me replying with the same. As soon as I stopped initiating phone calls and get-togethers, the friendship dried up.

Donna had disappointed me deeply, but I realized upon reflection I had set myself up for it. When she told me she was not a good friend, I had not listened. I had settled for a one-sided relationship from the beginning, never expecting reciprocity—an old habit leftover from my childhood.

Fortunately, she also did me a good turn: that text opened my eyes. I deserved better. I deserved friends who had my back, valued my time, and sought my company as often as I sought theirs. I decided to edit out all my one-sided relationships by looking for patterns over time.

Did I do all the initiating? If yes, I stepped back and considered each situation. Was this the relationship's usual pattern or a new development? Did the person have a new baby, an ill parent, or a demanding new job? If so, I cut them some slack. Even the best friends do not always have the bandwidth to nurture relationships outside of their immediate families, however they might want to.

Sometimes long-term friendships require us to forgive each other over and over, but sometimes we need to ask ourselves if the friendship has simply run its course. I decided that if a friend only called when they wanted something or only talked about their own problems without asking about my life, I would ask, "Does this this relationship nourish me?"

If not, I moved on.

Sometimes, we form strong bonds when we share an experience with another person, like Donna and I did. But once the experience ends, those friendships can shrink. I have had scores of friends in graduate school, parenting groups, and different workplaces who impacted my life significantly, but as circumstances changed, our relationships grew less intense or fell away. Seasonal friendships are no less powerful or important just because they do not last a lifetime.

Self-editing my connections had a profound effect on my life. Understanding what was wrong and why it was happening was only the first step. To actually feel better, I had to not only recognize what the problem was, I had to create a plan to change and follow through with it. As soon as I realized I could choose to create distance or closeness in my relationships without discussing it with the other person, I felt an empowered sense of freedom.

Manage Expectations

My siblings and I always tried to do something nice for Mother's Day. The few times we missed the mark, my mother felt wounded and withdrew in silence, making the day unpleasant for everyone.

As my kids entered kindergarten, I vowed to make Mother's Day easy for them and pleasant for me, so I devised a plan. "I want two things," I told them. "A handmade, heartfelt card, and a meal I do not make or clean up after."

My request evolved into a beautiful tradition: we would go to our favorite—not fancy, not Mother's Day-crowded—Vietnamese restaurant, and then go bowling at a completely empty alley. The tradition has survived my boys growing up and leaving the house. I still savor and save their exquisite letters, and I love eating at any interesting off-the-path ethnic restaurant. By communicating my preferences, I made it easy for my family to meet my expectations for a happy Mother's Day.

When People Let You Down

Disappointment averted. But it is not always that easy.

Sometimes, my frustrations stemmed from my own completely unrealistic expectations. I used to assume my loved ones—especially my children—would anticipate what I wanted. For example, when I arrived home after a long work trip and found the house a mess, I would experience a cascade of irritation, distress, and disappointment.

Once I took stock of the situation, I reminded myself that no one was actively trying to hurt or annoy me. My boys simply did not care about the house, and my husband was too busy with his own concerns to deal with it.

When I realized I was repeatedly setting myself up for disappointment with my own uncommunicated or unreasonable expectations, I created a plan to ask myself two questions to help me exit my superhighway to resentment:

Have I communicated what I want?

Is what I am asking for reasonable?

I had never specifically told the boys how I wanted the house to look when I got home, but asking them to clean up before my arrival was not unreasonable. I began calling an hour early to remind them, "Please clean up before I get there."

That released my own ill intentions, which I had been projecting on my family, communicated what I wanted and expected, and remedied the issue. Recognition, plan, follow-through.

Choosing Wellness

No matter how aware I am, friends and family will disappoint me—and I will disappoint them. That is just life. But I can enjoy life resentment-free if I edit my expectations and take responsibility for my own needs and communications.

Managing expectations, releasing disappointment, and avoiding resentment are all key to choosing wellness.

11 WORRY IS SELF-INFLICTED SUFFERING

When I first learned that my sister Ellen's two-year-old son had been diagnosed with HIV, I knew the prognosis was grim. Both she and her husband would end up dying from AIDS—an agonizing disease—within a few years.

But "Joshua" managed to stay well. He spent long parts of his summers with my husband and I as he grew up. We loved him deeply.

That love came bundled with outsized worry. Every single time I saw my nephew, I thought it would be the last. When he started kindergarten, I thought he would not make it to third grade. Then, when he started third grade, I felt sure he would not make it to fifth. On and on it went.

Every time he came down with a sniffle, I convinced myself this was it. So of course, I overindulged him.

Joshua came along on a family trout-fishing expedition when he was eight. He had spent his whole life in the city, and I wanted him to have the "nature experience" of catching a fish. Unfortunately, the fish were not biting that day. Operating from a place of "final wishes" and "only chances," I found a fish farm that guaranteed success: the owner threw bait into a pond and the fish swarmed. Within ten minutes, my nephew caught as many fish.

I gave him instant gratification over patience and skill, which was really bad parenting. Yet I could not stop. His horrific illness haunted me. I knew in my heart he faced the same long, excruciating, inevitable death I had witnessed my sister go through. Every time he coughed, I imagined his sad funeral. I thought about how I could possibly get through it, what I would say, how we would move away from the grave.

My worry clouded every aspect of my life.

When Joshua turned ten, the first HIV antiretroviral drugs became widely available for those who could afford it. They dramatically improved his prognosis—but not my anxiety. In fact, they actually heightened it.

When he came to visit that summer, as usual, I monitored his medication, as usual. He took up to twenty pills a day, but I found them all in the trash. "I can't swallow all those pills and capsules," he confessed. "I pretend to gulp them down, then when I'm alone, I spit them out."

Crazed with worry and determined to get the medication into him, I spent the next week forcing him to practice over and over until he could proficiently swallow his pills.

Worry is Self-Inflicted Suffering

But even that did not allay my fears. I simply could not talk myself down from worrying.

Eventually, Joshua graduated from high school, went onto college, and married his high-school sweetheart.

I could not find the words to toast him at his wedding. Despite his obvious good health and longevity, I had never thought he would live that long—and with such a high degree of wellbeing!

Ten years later, he and his wife decided to have a child. Thanks to ongoing research, Joshua's HIV is now nondetectable, so he will probably live long enough to teach his own children and grandchildren how to fish—without resorting to a fish farm.

And he will not pass the infection on to his children the way it had been passed onto him from his parents.

Through all those decades of worry, it never once occurred to me that new treatments would change HIV from a death-sentence disease into a manageable chronic illness that would let my nephew live a long and fruitful life. Instead, I had latched onto a catastrophic future—one that never came.

Worry Is Not Fear

Fear is a primal response to danger; it triggers an adrenaline release and energizes us to act. Fear is nature's built-in protection emotion. My fear about Joshua's health prodded me to help him learn how to swallow his pills.

Choosing Wellness

Worry comes from the Old English wyrgan, which meant "strangle," and the root definition still holds. We have mental distress about something anticipated, which strangles our wellbeing. Worry or anxiety is toxic, not protective. Worry does not move us to action; instead it paralyzes us in anticipation of potential or imagined danger. Anxiety is not about what is happening now but about what could happen, what might happen, what maybe will possibly happen, sometime, at some later date. Obsessing over Joshua's imminent death—which was never imminent at all—neither altered the course of his disease or, in fact, affected him at all.

It merely cast a pall over my precious time with him.

Worry did not prepare me for disappointment or grief. I practiced my nephew's funeral a number of times, but that did not inure me to the pain of losing him—I felt it every time. I just made myself suffer for no good reason.

I had deluded myself about Joshua. Worry may have made me feel more connected to him, but it was an unhealthy, corrosive connection. I had told myself that worrying would prevent bad things from happening.

It did not. It cannot. And yes, despite believing I could not stop myself from worrying, I have learned that I can.

Worry is an emotion, so like with any other emotion, I have taught myself to notice when it creeps in, acknowledge its presence, and ask myself a series of questions to assess my feelings:

Worry is Self-Inflicted Suffering

- What am I worried about?
- Is there anything I can do to positively impact the situation?
- If there is nothing I can do, how can I focus my attention on something else?
- Do I need to admit my powerlessness?
- Am I anticipating failure?
- Am I letting my own concerns impede someone else's growth or autonomy?
- What are other possible outcomes beside the ones I am imagining?

And as I worked on how to really listen, I learned what worry sounds like: "I don't want you to get hurt, so I don't want you to—

… learn how to drive."

… study abroad."

… live alone when you're eighty."

Those emotional responses naturally lead to conflict: my wants and needs against the other person's independence. When someone tells me about a problem they are having, I have learned to not impulsively try to restrict their autonomy, but rather to respect it. I recognize their right to make their own decisions—and their own mistakes. So now my responses are: "I understand you want to—

… learn to drive. What kind of agreement should we make about it?"

… study abroad. Let's talk about how and when."

Choosing Wellness

… live alone when you're eighty. How will we know when you need help?"

I only prepared for disaster throughout Joshua's entire childhood, so I never noticed the miracle unfolding before me: The child who was never sick. The new drug treatments. The boy who grew into a kind and thoughtful man. The man who became a father.

How I wish I could tell my younger self: "Love him. Enjoy your life. There's nothing to fear, so STOP WORRYING and look for the good!"

12 MY SWAN DIVE

I had just switched to buying organic milk to shield myself from pesticides and antibiotics. Yet, every night I drank wine until I passed out.

I asked myself, "Would my teenage self be proud of who I am today?" The dichotomy was startling. My sixteen-year-old self had dreamed of being a nurse since age eleven. She had clarity about who she wanted to be: a person who values health. She went on to fulfill her nursing dreams. By twenty-one, she had earned her RN, quit smoking, and begun a daily exercise regimen. By twenty-four, she achieved success as a nurse practitioner in a major academic health center.

Now, two decades later, she—I—was proud of everything I had fought to accomplish, everything I did to help others achieve and sustain their own health. But every morning, I woke with a hangover; every morning I promised myself to "cut down" or "just have two" that evening. Every bad hangover made me vow to switch from wine to brandy, gin, beer, or even whiskey, alcohol I disliked. Sometimes I even tried drinking just on weekends. Still, no matter my intentions, I lost my resolve in a new bottle of wine every day at five o'clock in the afternoon.

No, my younger me was not at all proud of who I had become. I had no integrity.

For the most part, I hid this daily habit well. Anybody looking at me on the outside would see a veneer of success. Anybody looking at me closely would sense something was wrong. Nobody in my life was confronting me about this, which speaks to my stealth in hiding and covering it.

Recognizing my organic-milk hypocrisy was not enough motivation to make me change my behavior, though. I did not find that impetus until my eight-year-old son woke me to make breakfast one morning. He eyed me with obvious concern as I stumbled around the kitchen, barely able to function.

"You look beautiful today, Mom," he said.

I caught my breath. My little boy was trying to make me feel better the only way he knew how. He clearly saw the truth I had not faced.

And it broke me. I stood at the refrigerator, hungover as I had been every morning for longer than I wanted to admit, and I could not tolerate myself another minute. I had sworn I would not turn into my mother, yet here I was, creating the same kind of alcoholic home I grew up in, where shame and fear are permanent residents, yet everyone pretends all is well and the lack of security remains unspoken.

I had betrayed the sixteen-year-old me who vowed to construct a different future. More importantly, I was betraying my children and husband with those broken vows. I had to find my way back to the person who deeply valued health. I just did not know how.

I thought about that Abe Lincoln biography I had read—the one where I learned his secret about writing angry letters but not sending them. His struggle to hold together a warring nation resonated deeply with me because I, too, was a house divided. My two identities—the passionate health expert and the self-loathing lush—were at constant war.

I wanted to be true to myself—but I did not want to give up alcohol. I liked it too much. It made me numb. It relieved all my anxieties. It buried my past horrors, so I did not have to face them.

Of course, it also gave me a daily sense of impending doom, since I was sure I would be found out any moment: the other shoe would drop, the gig would be up, something terrible would happen. This was not the kind of anxiety I felt about my nephew's health; this was real fear about being arrested, forced into rehab, and losing my nursing license, not to mention my kids, my marriage, and my dignity. Drinking put me on a giant swan dive into a dark place where I could not lower my standards fast enough to keep up with my degrading behavior.

I had toyed with the idea of quitting for a long time. I even talked about it with people close to me. The heavy drinkers laughed. "You don't have a problem," they scoffed.

"Buy an eighty-dollar bottle of wine, pour yourself a glass, and relax after the kids fall asleep," a soon-fired therapist advised.

My primary-care physician waved her hand dismissively. "Your liver-function tests are all normal. Just cut down."

Even my husband, who often worked evenings and weekends, denied I had a drinking problem. "Just slow down," he said. "Pace yourself."

But a recovering-alcoholic friend offered the best advice: "Set yourself a limit. If you cannot stick to it, you have an addiction."

I already knew I could not keep a self-imposed limit. With the Lincoln metaphor ringing in my head, I had the impulse to chase the metaphor to its conclusion. I searched the internet: "How do civil wars end?"

Amazingly, crushing defeat of one side resulted in permanent peace for the warring nation far more often than compromise, I discovered in a Harvard study. There was my truth, my radical acceptance: if I wanted to end my own civil war, I had to conquer my drinking head-on. There was to be no compromise, no cutting down, no half measures.

My Swan Dive

My identity as a health-expert had to crush my alcohol induced self-loathing. Swift defeat was the only answer. I attended my first recovery meeting that same day.

First Meeting

I climbed a long staircase with a light at the top, shaking with fear, defeat, and inner hatred. People sat in a circle of chairs. They welcomed me and asked me why I was there.

"I'm worried about my drinking," I said with embarrassment—and then the tears started. I told them everything between heaving sobs.

No one interrupted me. No one judged me.

When I finished, someone else shared their story. Then another person. And another. Listening to everyone around the circle speak from their hearts about their alcohol problems and sobriety was somehow calming. I even felt a tiny glimmer of hope.

Afterwards, the man who had sat next to me said, "I hid my problem, too. I've been where you are. I understand. I stashed alcohol in my janitor's cart for years before I became sober. Let me give you some advice."

"Okay."

"Go home and pray. Don't drink tonight. Come back tomorrow."

"That's it?"

"That's it. Go home and pray. Don't drink tonight. Come back tomorrow."

I went home, but I did not pray. I did not trust God or anything else I could not see. But I walked out to my backyard and stood before the only altar I knew—our old oak tree.

"Please help me not drink," I pleaded.

I did not reach for a wine bottle that night.

I went back the next day and talked to the same man. He gave me the same instructions: "Don't drink tonight. Seek help from your higher power. Come to tomorrow's meeting."

It felt a little ridiculous to hold heartfelt conversations with a tree, but somehow it worked. I returned a third day and received more advice: "Don't try to understand it. Just do it."

By the fourth day, I felt giddy. I was living without alcohol for the first time in years.

On day five, I came clean to my husband about everything: the drinking, the hiding, the recovery meetings. "I plan to do everything they say for three months without question," I told him.

"I don't think you're an alcoholic," he repeated. "But if you feel you have to do this, then I support you."

Radical Acceptance

I actually attended ninety meetings in ninety days, not my planned thirty in thirty. I found a sponsor (a person with solid recovery from addiction who closely helps others get and stay sober) and went through the twelve steps. It took a long time to admit alcohol is my kryptonite, but when I did, that radical acceptance completely overhauled my life, changing my thoughts, my career, my identity, and my friends. It even changed what I do in my free time.

That janitor saved my life. I now fully inhabit my sober identity.

Still, I remind myself daily that I have a chronic progressive illness which, if I am not vigilant, will first isolate and then kill me. I view alcohol the way someone with a horrific seafood allergy views shellfish: one taste and it is all over. One sip of wine will trigger an intense craving no matter what the consequences.

That truth lives in my bones and courses through my blood.

And now that I have radically accepted my circumstances, I know my sixteen-year-old-self would be damn proud of who I became.

13 THREE GENERATIONS OF DESTRUCTION

When my oldest son and I arrived at a preschool gym class, I got annoyed when he refused to remove his shoes to join the class. "Look at those other kids," I told him. "They're taking off their shoes. Do what they're doing."

Hearing the idiocy of my own words broke through my irritation, and my brain suddenly fast-forwarded. I imagined twelve years from now when I could hear my adolescent son say, "All the kids at school smoke weed. Everybody's doing it."

Flash of insight: I am parenting like my mother!

Since my mother had pushed conformity, I unconsciously defaulted to the only parenting model I ever knew. But as soon as I recognized that, I also recognized I did not want my children to blindly follow someone else's script—not even mine. I wanted to affirm their autonomy and help them gain a strong, unshakable sense of themselves that would steady them through adolescence's impulsivity and peer pressure.

I started taking Parent Encouragement Program (PEP) classes based on developmental-psychologist Alfred Adler's theories. He developed a framework for parenting that promoted raising kids with a high degree of social interest, self-regulation, competence and belonging. Over the next four years I made a stunning discovery: parenting is not intuitive.

No one is born with insights into child psychology. No one "naturally" has the skills to handle developmental challenges. If I did not actively seek best-parenting practices, I would be limited to what I picked up from family and friends.

In one class, I learned anger often masks other emotions. I might lash out over spilt milk, for example, but the milk is not the real issue—I might be concerned about my husband's behavior or work stress. As with so many other wellness strategies, I needed to get under my anger and discover its root cause. My first assignment: "Describe a common anger situation with your kids."

My sons were eight and six, so I immediately thought of bedtime. My husband often worked late, so it was up to me to do the dinner-bath-teeth-brushing-reading routine with the boys. But once tucked into bed, they would not settle down and go to sleep. They horsed around, asked for water, or begged for more stories.

Eventually, I would lose my temper.

Every night.

"Describe how you felt."

Tired.

"Does the anger match the situation?"

"NO!" I scratched on the worksheet. While irritation or frustration might have been appropriate for these bedtime antics, I felt more of a slow, seething rage.

"List every reason for being angry."

I filled in the obvious: "I'm tired, it's my time, I'm spent."

"Why are you so angry in this situation?"

"I feel played and manipulated," I wrote. "The children are inconsiderate and don't think about anyone but themselves."

I stopped writing. That last response did not feel true. Selfishness did not fit with my anger. I had to mull over why my anger did not match the situation. I set the worksheet aside and went to bed thinking about that question.

Later that night, I bolted upright in bed, gasping with the real answer: I was jealous of my oldest son!

I knew it was true because I burned with embarrassment. My anger masked my jealousy, an emotion I was too ashamed to admit. It came into my full consciousness and I could see it.

Sitting with this truth over the next few days, I thought about why I envied my son. Everything came easily to him. He brought home report cards filled with As, yet I knew he often did his homework on the bus. A naturally gifted athlete, he excelled on the basketball court, and all his easy successes gave him confidence and made him secure with himself. To top it off, he had the material, emotional, and logistical support—from me and his father!—to pursue what he liked.

He was a happy, unconditionally loved kid with a childhood I could not help comparing to my own.

Everything came hard to me. I was a weak, scrappy student with an undiagnosed learning disorder. I never experienced abundance with food, clothing, school supplies, safety, or love. I had no special talent to feed my confidence. I had failed at bowling, the only sport I ever tried out for.

My mother was an angry, sometimes violent alcoholic throughout my childhood. Even when sober, she would lash out with unpredictable rage, unless we had company at the house—then she became a wonderful, animated, funny person who everyone adored. Even me. Life would have been easier to navigate if she passed out at four o'clock every day, but I could not even count on that.

When I shared this ugly insight with my husband, he said, "I've always thought your mother was jealous of you. The first time I met her, I noticed how she kept trying to direct my attention from you to her. She dominated every conversation, talking about incidental things that did not mean anything to me. She was always like that; I saw the same thing over and over again."

I had no idea that dynamic existed—but once he pointed it out, I remembered my grandmother criticizing my mother for everything: how she parented, how she kept house, how she was lazy and wasteful. Grandma had lived through the depression, so maybe her huge power struggle with her own daughter stemmed from the same thing: jealousy. She probably resented my mother's "easy" life, just as my mother resented how I had pulled mine together when she could not—and I resented my son for enjoying the easy path my husband and I had given him.

With one anger worksheet, I discovered a pattern going back at least three generations, if not much, much further. Sudden clarity hit me with an enormous jolt: my grandmother, my mother, and I all envied our kids, and so unwittingly competed with and undermined them.

I felt heartbroken about my mother. She had never reined in her anger, drinking, or verbal and physical abusiveness. She had never taken responsibility for the harm she inflicted on my siblings and me. She must have felt guilty and resentful and frustrated and disappointed every day of her life. At the same time, I was grateful my son had me, an emotionally tuned-in mother who did not model extreme dysfunction as a normal lifestyle. I wanted and expected I would have a lifelong friendly relationship with him, which I certainly never had with my mother.

From that moment, my bedtime anger vanished. I started watching for destructive past-interaction patterns whenever something came up. Then I would reset my intentions and change my behavior, making my conscious living a wellness choice.

Now when I look at my son, I marvel at what he has become: a secure, confident, nonconformist person. He had and is having an incredible life, doing things that, yes, sometimes raise a tinge of envy. But now when that happens, I just smile. I am so grateful for my ever-growing self-awareness, which is helping me yank out my own destructive roots of envy, live in choice, and be the parent I always wanted to be.

14 MEDITATION

Early in my recovery when I was in my forties, friends told me I needed a spiritual intervention.

They were not just casual friends; "Eva" and "Alex" and I had been in practice together when I was a nurse practitioner in a primary-care clinic in my early twenties. We had shared an office and helped each other through various emotional trials: Eva's marriage to a man with grown kids after years of being single; Alex's complicated pregnancy and miscarriage; my sister's addiction and death.

Both women were about ten years older than me and had done deep work on their own self-awareness, spiritual growth, and healing, so I valued them as professional mentors as well as personal friends. We had fallen out of touch with each other, as will happen when people find other jobs and get busy with life. But one day, after more than a decade of little contact, the three of us met for lunch.

Meditation

When it was my turn to update them on my life, I ranted about a troubling family member and complained about my job.

"You seem really angry," Eva commented.

Alex nodded. "If you're really done with that family member," she said calmly, "then why are you still fixating on her? Be done. And if your work does not suit you. . . well, what are you doing about it?"

Their candor was like a punch in the face.

"Eileen, this seething anger isn't like you," Alex continued. "What's going on?"

"I know a counselor," Eva offered. "She teaches meditation and helps people develop spiritually."

I shook my head. "Thanks, but I don't believe in anything I can't see. I'm already in a recovery program and rejected its "higher power" spirituality. I'm not interested in organized religion, not even Buddhism."

"But this counselor just helps you focus on how to quiet your mind. It's not a religious thing at all! It's more of a mind-body thing. A wellness thing," she finished.

"Well. . . okay," I gave in. "I'll give her a call."

I set an appointment for a few days after my son's birthday party at a premier sports and recreational complex. I signed a contract with the facility, sent out the invites, arranged for transportation, and had each parent sign a waiver. With my husband working the day of, I would be responsible for all the children, both at the site and getting them home.

Choosing Wellness

No problem, I thought. I can handle fifteen kids for two hours, especially if they are playing indoor soccer. Besides, I want my son's eighth birthday to be special.

I was fine watching the kids play soccer for about forty-five minutes, despite the blaring music, screeching whistles, and ball thumping from the other basketball courts, batting cages, and indoor soccer fields. Then the party organizer herded the boys into a dingy, filthy room to serve them horrendously bad pizza, sugary drinks, and cake.

I sang the happy birthday song through gritted teeth.

Then the organizer gave each kid tokens for the arcade games and they immediately dispersed in every direction. Keeping track of them was impossible. I lost it.

I attacked the organizer, viciously detailing the hell hole she worked in. Completely out of control, I refused to be comforted, assured, or soothed. The poor girl did not know what to do with my rage.

Not my best moment.

The next day, I wrote a two-page apology to her and resolved to keep my appointment with the spiritual counselor, Robbins. I told her about the incident almost before I sat down in her office.

"I'm ashamed of what I did," I said. "I don't want to be this person. I don't want my anger to ambush me like that."

Robbins nodded. "You had to deal with a lot of stress before the party even started," she pointed out. "Is it possible that working out all the logistics might have touched off some resentment?"

"Yes," I said. "That sounds about right."

"Then you might've already had a chip on your shoulder when you walked through the door," Robbins said. "The noise didn't help; it could've triggered some low-level irritation, which then ticked up when you noticed the filthy room and the bad food. By then, you were probably furious with yourself for planning a party experience that went against your own values and didn't in any way live up to your idea of a birthday celebration—though it probably was a blast for the eight-year-olds. And since you weren't aware all this was going on," Robbins went on, "you felt ambushed."

Wow, I thought. This woman totally gets me!

"You can learn to pay attention to what's happening inside your head, your heart, and your body before anger erupts," Robbins said. "You can learn to notice thoughts and feelings like an outside observer, so you don't get caught up in them. That's what meditation does for you. Want to try it for just five minutes?"

"Yes, please!"

"Sit in an upright, alert position and close your eyes," she instructed. "Now, just pay attention to the sensation of your breath moving in and out of your nose or lungs. Your thoughts will wander.

"That's okay. That's what the mind does. Gently guide it back to the breath.

Choosing Wellness

"Imagine your mind as a toddler. You direct it to the park, but she sees a bug and stops. Let her go ahead and look at the bug, and then nudge her back toward the park, or, in this case, back toward the breath. Keep doing that over and over without judging yourself."

Like most people who meditate for the first time, I discovered my brain was more like a hyperactive toddler on a sugar high. My thoughts danced away from my breathing every two seconds. Chasing after them got me lost down one rabbit hole after another, but once I realized what was happening, I brought my attention back to my breath.

I felt calmer even after just five minutes.

"I want to continue this practice," I told Robbins.

"Good. Then I recommend you join one of my meditation groups."

At first it was torture to sit still and focus, but after several months of weekly sessions and daily practice, I entered a peaceful space where the outside world disappeared. I lost all notion of place and time and felt deeply relaxed.

Robbins also helped me discover how to call out my best self, to be aware of my body, to notice the first sign of chest tightening or nasal flaring as my personal early warning system. Pulling from a huge range of sources, she helped me practice self-compassion, kindness, consciousness, and connectivity.

She introduced me to a spiritual energy I couldn't see but could ask for help anytime or anyplace I needed it—and she did not insist I call it God, or believe in metaphysics, or understand the zero-point field. She wanted her clients to feel a strong spiritual bond to something outside ourselves so we could move toward loving kindness not only to others, but to ourselves—and move away from feeling we must handle everything on our own, which leads to worry, despair, and obsessive thoughts.

I eventually learned how to drop into a meditative state on my own. It is not, as some people think, a zombie trance, but rather a peaceful consciousness, an alpha-wave state of stillness that allows wisdom in. If I need help accepting a situation or guidance on how to proceed with something, I ask for it beforehand and then see what comes up during my meditation. Other times I simply sit still and let thoughts pass. Without fail, the practice leaves me with a deeper sense of serenity, something I had never wanted, experienced, or even known about until midlife.

While I am not perfect at it and sometimes miss days, I am a better version of myself since learning this practice. My old mind could not stop revenge fantasies or dark, obsessive thoughts. My new mind can. Meditation is like a superpower that makes me less reactive to whatever is happening around me. I am calmer, more thoughtful, and more intentional in what I do and where I place my energy.

I rarely experience emotional ambushes now. I no longer sleepwalk through choices or get blindsided by my own reactions; research shows long-term meditators lose their startle reflex. I can change my own brain architecture. We are not at the mercy of primitive wiring with its hypersensitive focus on negative stimuli that keeps us constantly stressed.

When I learned to quiet my mind, I gained agency, or command, over myself and where I placed my energies. Meditation not only cured my soul sickness; it was a gamechanger in my pursuit of high-level wellness.

15 DARK TEACHERS

My good friend "Sandy" and I first connected when her three boys and my two sons played together in the neighborhood. We had everything in common: We were working mothers. We enjoyed yoga. We loved long walks. We co-hosted a mother-son book club.

And we shared a glass or two several evenings a week.

I admired Sandy's lust for life. When she once said, "Hey, let's take the kids to New York!" We caught the train from DC, where we lived, to Manhattan, where Sandy guided everyone through Chinatown. She showed us how to find great knock-off sunglasses and introduced us to the best dumplings on the planet. She even taught us how to scavenge for inexpensive tickets to a super-hero Broadway show. Needless to say, the kids were thrilled. Sandy gave us a love for NYC that my boys and I carry to this day.

Choosing Wellness

Another time, she and I left the kids with our husbands and flew to London. We saw six plays in four days, including a one-woman pub show, where the performer invited the audience to give her feedback on that night's new material. I had no idea what to say to her, but Sandy had been immersed in the performance and was so insightful, she knew exactly what to tell the actress. The two of them had a lively conversation afterwards, while I stood to the side, feeling lucky to witness such an upbeat, fascinating exchange.

Sandy fit in everywhere. A good listener, she never judged. Instead, she always made people laugh and feel at ease.

She also matched me drink for drink, so when I started wondering if I had a problem, she was the first person I asked. I valued her perspective because she was so smart in ways I was not: a whiz at math, an avid reader, an engineer who had earned her degree from Carnegie Mellon.

After listening carefully on one of our long walks, she acknowledged my feelings, but ultimately dismissed my concerns. "You're just stressed," she assured me.

I desperately wanted her to be right.

But the night before my son told me I looked beautiful while i was stumbling around in the kitchen, Sandy and I drank far more than usual at an outdoor Bonnie Raitt concert.

I only remember parts of the evening, but I clearly recall her getting violently ill.

Dark Teachers

I did not tell Sandy I was going to a recovery meeting that next afternoon when I asked her to watch my kids. I did not want her to try to discourage me from going. I thought about asking her to come with me, but at my core I knew this was a solo journey.

We did not meet for a drink that night, when I spent the evening begging my oak tree for help. I do not remember exactly when I told her I was experimenting with sobriety, but our yoga, walks, and joint-family vacations slowly came to an end. So did the New York weekends. We drifted apart even more when I tried to talk with her about recovery. At first, she just shut down our conversations. Eventually, she shut me out completely.

As the years passed, Sandy grew increasingly isolated. I stopped seeing her in her yard; we never ran into each other at school functions or while running errands. I did see her kids at my house more and more frequently, though, as they were still close friends with my sons. They would tell me, "She lies about everything," or, "She's drinking all of the time." I offered to bring them to support meetings, but they did not want to take that step.

Eventually, Sandy sent me a letter from a twenty-eight-day rehab program she was doing. When she returned home, she told me she was attending early-morning recovery meetings every day.

Everything is fine, I thought. She is following a parallel path to mine. Admittedly, it did not feel the same as my recovery, but that is the whole point of a solo journey. We gave each other lots of space.

A few years after Sandy's rehab, her husband called out of the blue. "She's been in the hospital for a month with advanced liver failure," he said. "I found empty bottles hidden all over the house, and her credit card statement shows daily charges from the local liquor store.

"Eileen, she's been drinking half a gallon of vodka a day."

He told me that she was home for Christmas, and he needed somebody to help take care of her so he could attend his oldest son's college graduation out of town.

I had not been to Sandy's house in years, and I was shocked at how much her health had deteriorated.

Looking up at me from the pillows, she said, "I know. I have a mountain to climb. But I'm gonna fix this."

We talked about her drinking in an open and honest way for the first time. She talked about how alcoholism had damaged not only her, but her family who she loved deeply. That made me hopeful, despite her appearance. I thought she had hit her bottom, as alcoholics need to do before they can really pursue recovery.

"I know I can never drink again," she said. "I'm ready and determined to battle my addiction."

"I'm on your team and your biggest cheerleader," I assured her, holding her jaundiced hands. "I want you to succeed. I want you back. Your life can be mended and made whole. You can go back to being your amazing you."

Dark Teachers

We spent many hours together those few days. I told her recovery stories I had seen and heard: People whose lives were in shambles. Prison sentences. Estranged families. Every betrayal and humiliating act I could think of. "Healing and reconciliation happened all the time," I kept saying. "You can do this."

I met one of Sandy's sponsors during a visit.

"No one realized she was still drinking," the sponsor told me. "She even received her one-year-sober medallion."

"So, what happened?"

"Someone smelled alcohol on her breath and asked her about it. She left the recovery meeting and never came back."

Sandy was re-admitted to the hospital within days. But her liver failure was already too advanced; her body would not last until she could get a transplant. She was in hospice within a week.

Five days later, she was gone. She was only fifty-two years old.

I was devastated, furious, despondent, and mostly heartbroken. My beautiful, brilliant friend had drank herself to death.

In *It's a Wonderful Life*, an angel lets suicidal George Bailey, overwhelmed with financial problems, see what his community would have been like without him.

Sandy was that same glimpse into my own life. I do not know why I found the strength to face my alcoholism while she did not. No one knows why one person can and another cannot. If anyone ever solves this mystery, it will alleviate horrendous suffering around the world. I only know that what we do not want is a powerful motivator to achieve what we do want.

A Turkish proverb says, "No matter how far you've gone on the wrong road, turn around."

I agree—but that is not always the full truth when dealing with addiction.

Sandy was my dark teacher. I am incredibly sad for losing her and how she left. My life depends on remembering this.

16 EMOTIONAL VAMPIRES

I first encountered the term "emotional vampire" in Judith Orloff's *Emotional Freedom*. It clicked with me; I definitely knew people who sucked the life out of me. In fact, I was related to several.

I have a helping complex, so I often get consumed by resentment and exhaustion without realizing I am being manipulated and drained by the emotional vampire I am trying to help. My sister Ellen was an emotional vampire.

So was my mother.

There are several flavors of emotional vampire, they show up differently, but will always leave us feeling drained and depleted.

The Victim

Everybody who met my mother loved her. She was gregarious and outgoing and had a huge laugh. She once did a survey of the proper way to hang paper towels and toilet paper (she believed "over" was the only right way), so for months, anybody who entered our house had to demo how they hung paper towels. She made a big running joke of it, finally declaring the "under" hangers had brain defects and needed treatment.

She was quirky, funny, self-deprecating, and practical. She always brought gifts to all six of her children's teachers in the beginning of the year so we would "reap the benefit" of her generosity.

A complicated woman with a larger-than-life personality, she lost her spleen in childhood due to a clotting disorder, and people treated her as "sickly" from then on. No one expected much from or for her; no one expected her to make it to adulthood.

She made it.

When she married at twenty-two, she was told she would not be able to bear children.

She had six.

Perhaps all those contradictions are what conspired to make her into a self-pitying, textbook "victim" who blamed her misfortunes on the world and took no responsibility for her own actions, emotional landscape, or life difficulties—privately, that is. Publicly, no one ever knew she embraced victimhood or thought the world actively conspired against her. "These things just happen to me," she would say bravely. "I don't know why."

And her friends would believe her, nodding with sympathy.

Victim vampires complain frequently, yet flatly and swiftly reject solutions with a "yeah...but" response. Since they do not really want to change—in fact, they see no reason why they should—interacting with them is one-directional; I would continually give, but she would not or could not receive.

Obese, my mother also suffered from congestive heart failure (CHF), a chronic, progressive condition wherein the heart cannot pump sufficient oxygen and blood to the whole body. It can shorten a person's lifespan, but people can live with it for decades as long as they vigilantly monitor their symptoms and take care of themselves.

My mother had CHF for over ten years, so she knew she could manage it by controlling her salt intake and watching her weight. Whenever her legs, ankles, or feet swelled up, she had to increase her diuretic medication to eliminate the buildup so her lungs would not fill with fluid and her heart would not have trouble pumping blood.

If CHF is not controlled, it can be fatal.

Despite knowing all this, she drove seven hours with swollen legs from Connecticut to Washington, DC to attend a cousin's wedding. She did not want to take the time to increase her medication and wait for the edema to go down because, she explained, "I'd have had to stop every fifteen minutes!"

Instead, she showed up at my door two days early, out of breath and barely able to walk. And she devoured a salty chicken dish a family friend brought over, never thinking about her already swollen legs.

She woke me at two o'clock that morning complaining of chest pain and difficulty breathing. I took her to the emergency room, where she received an IV diuretic and passed a liter of fluid.

She immediately felt much better, of course, but we had all spent the night in the ER.

On the way home, I asked, "How are you tracking your water weight and sodium intake?"

"I don't know what you mean," she said. "Nobody ever told me I have to weigh myself or avoid salt. Besides," she grumbled, "how did I know the dish was salty?"

She did not want to know. She had to know to watch her weight and salt intake because we had that conversation many times as well. But to her, remarkably, the ER visit was a random event, something that "happened to her" completely unconnected to her actions.

I was still at the point where I thought my job was to fix, fix, fix my family, friends, and, of course, patients. So instead, I offered ideas about how to avoid future ER visits.

A true victim, she dismissed each one with a, "That's a good idea, but…" excuse.

My resentment boiled; I was more invested in solving my mother's problems than she was! This is an early warning sign. I had not yet realized I had any agency in the matter, but I did know to read my resentment as a warning sign, and to pause and consider my own actions. That night in the ER may have been just another "thing that happens to me," for my mother, but it was a vital turning point for me. The recognition hit me like a thunderbolt: I was over-invested in my mother!

From then on, I needed to pause and triage whenever I dealt with her.

Triage is the sorting process medical professionals use to decide which patients require urgent attention, which can wait, and how—even if—they can help someone. This same concept can used by anyone to sort the challenging people in our lives. If we triage a vampire—be it victim, know-it-all, downer, or conflict-generator, or the grande dame of all, a narcissist—we know not to deplete our time and energy on them. We can resist our urge to give advice, try to fix who they are, or control any of it. We can let the responsibility lie where it belongs: with them.

Thinking of my mother along those lines required a sharp mindset shift. It meant I would no longer carry her burden in any way. I would radically accept how she lived, so I would not do or commit myself to anything that would make me resentful. Had I acted to protect myself instead of my mother at two am that morning, I would have checked her into the ER and gone home to bed.

Easy to say, hard to do.

The Know-it-all

Unlike victims, who never know why things happen to them, the know-it-all is fused to their own knowledge. Stuck in the past, they cherry pick facts to ensure they are always right. Since their ego cannot risk being wrong, they may pretend to listen when someone else talks, but their mind is closed to hearing other points of view. When challenged, they dig in to defend and protect their self-image as the smartest person in the room.

Just as victims are not interested in solutions, know-it-alls are not interested in learning.

Trying to have a genuine exchange with a know-it-all leaves me feeling diminished and drained, if not outright frustrated. When I triage this energy suck, I let them be right and create distance in the relationship. I create mental freedom by not investing so much.

The Downer

Downers search for negativity on a global scale.

They find fault with everything and everyone because whatever the problem may be, it is always out there somewhere, never within themselves. They also very seldom recognize kindness or take notice when something goes well.

Downers not only drain energy, their toxic cynicism can siphon away optimism, plunging us into such a negative state that we cannot focus on solutions, envision new possibilities, or even simply enjoy our day.

I stopped trying to cheer up downers or change their world view; the effort demands endless energy, too much time, and in the long run, accomplishes nothing. Now, when someone meets my hopeful outlook with a deluge of negativity or leaves me feeling dejected, I immediately seek an escape route. I am no longer compelled to play the role of cheerleader.

The Conflict/Drama Generator

Conflict/drama generators are more difficult to identify because their behavior pattern only shows up in long-term relationships. I would not call a co-worker who files a discrimination claim a conflict/drama generator, nor a neighbor who sues their contractor—unless they repeat those actions regularly, like my acquaintance who filed six personal-injury lawsuits!

Conflict/drama generators intentionally create chaos so they can feed off the adrenaline surges they create. Being around them can be exhilarating at first, but eventually they drain their supporters' spirit and goodwill, leaving everyone exhausted, bewildered, and battle fatigued. The only way I have ever figured out how to combat drama is to not get caught in others' drama in the first place. But if I do, as soon as I recognize the drain, I immediately release their burden, pull back, and watch the fireworks from a safe distance.

The Narcissist

Narcissism is a singularly distinct and malignant type of difficult emotional vampire, identifiable by four main pillars which are often an amalgam of victims, know-it-alls, and drama generators. Narcissists have: 1) enormous sense of grandiosity, 2) unbridled sense of entitlement, 3) a bottomless need for validation, and 4) a lack of empathy. They manipulate, lie, and gaslight to get what they want. There is no cure or treatment for narcissism, which is recognized by the American Psychiatric Association's Diagnostic and Statistical Manual of Mental Disorders (DSM 5) as a personality disorder.

People close to narcissists never feel they are doing enough—and they are right, since they cannot possibly measure up to the narcissist's constantly changing or expanding needs and desires. No matter how much we try, no matter what extent we go to please the narcissist in our life, we never will, we never can, gain their approval. No matter how much we give, they always need more, much more.

Narcissists are a destructive, wholly corrosive force of nature. They are crazy-making for intimate partners, co-workers, and anybody else close to them. Their ego needs can look like an addiction, as addicts might act like a narcissist sometimes, but that is not necessarily a permanent condition for them. If they enter a recovery process, the narcissism-from-addiction usually recedes, allowing them to develop healthy intimate relationships.

Triage is crucial, although tricky. Narcissists present as charming people, and they know how to use that charm as a weapon. Outsiders often see them as gracious, loving, and delightful, but those on the inside know that façade will vanish as soon as the door closes behind the last guest.

When I hear my clients rationalizing a relationship—"He's a great guy, except when…" "She's wonderful, except when…" "I love him, but I'm constantly walking on eggshells…"—We decide together if they are caught in a narcissist's tentacles.

Although my role is to help clients recognize the issues in their lives with my support and not my advice, I make an exception for people trapped in a narcissist's web. Stop playing their game right now. Set massive boundaries and cut off their food source: you, your generosity, your good heart—your own wellbeing. People close to narcissists eventually find their own health deteriorating. You must get out of their orbit by any means necessary.

Do not walk away—run!

If you cannot completely disengage, try "gray-rocking." When your narcissist tries to get attention, give them no reaction, offer them no appeasement. They will undoubtedly work even harder at that point to get a reaction, but you must remain a gray rock. Over time, they will look for another narcissist food source, and you can begin healing.

Triaging Vampires

I have a long history of being overinvested in other people's problems, so I learned to recognize when I am in dodgy territory. If I feel even a twinge of resentment—if what I am doing does not come from a place of love and generosity—I rein myself in.

If I am faced with a victim vampire, I disengage with a neutralizing, dead-end statement that gives the validation or pity they seek without taking any energy from me:

"You might be right."

"I see. Good to know."

"I'm sorry that happened to you. You poor thing."

When I have to deal with a know-it-all, I let them be right—it's what they want anyway—and then pivot to a more productive discussion:

"You are so correct. Now let's focus on solutions to the problem."

"You're right, that's how it has been done in the past. Now we're going to face the future differently."

"Good point! Now let's hear from others we haven't heard from yet."

I counter downer-vampire toxicity with:

"I have a place deep inside me that's sacred, and I work hard to keep it clean and free of darkness. I cannot have [gossip, negativity, unwanted criticism, drama, etc.] land on me."

Emotional Vampires

When a conflict/drama generator indirectly undermines me, I remind myself that they are adrenaline junkies, but I am not—nor do I need to be. I do not have to buy into their chaos. I can let them stew in their own juices without stirring the pot for them.

When I must deal with a narcissist socially or in the workplace, I deliberately choose to internally disengage. I flip on my gray-rock switch and move on as quickly as possible. I have already edited out all the narcissists in my personal life. Save yourself, for you cannot, no matter how much love, effort, money, or time you put in, save them.

Those of us naturally driven to help others will always struggle with turning our backs on emotional vampires until we learn to triage. This has been one of the hardest fought lessons of my life.

The Vampire in the Mirror

According to vampire lore, they do not appear in mirrors because they lack a soul. According to my own experience, vampires are incapable of self-reflection. Any honest attempt to ward off emotional vampires, therefore, must start with a crucial self-examination: Am I one?

Do I relish playing the victim?

We all indulge in self-pity at some point in our lives. It is a normal, almost unavoidable first response to devastating loss, life-threating illness, or unforeseen crisis. I do not know if humans are the only species that experiences self-pity; maybe its evolutionary benefit was the capacity for empathy. We can never know. But I do know that while other emotions serve us in some way, self-pity is entirely corrosive to those of us indulging in it and to everyone around us. Whatever the reason it first existed; it no longer serves us in modern life.

Wallowing in self-pity leaves me disempowered and disconnected to the love and people I need the most during a crisis or loss, so no, I do not relish playing the victim. I much prefer digging down to the root of my distress and taking positive action to fix it.

Do I feel threatened by disagreement, new knowledge, or other perspectives?

Being right all the time might feel empowering, but that is a self-deception. The know-it-all posture shuts out other people, spoils relationships, kills ideas, and makes personal growth impossible. We can love to learn, seek out other perspectives, and know that disagreement often leads to new awareness and growth. With intention and practice, knowledge or conflict need not be threatening

Do I suck the joy out of life?

Playing the perpetual killjoy may indicate depression— or just being unknowingly stuck in misery mode. As a nurse practitioner student, my fears and stress made me moody and irritable—I was a downer to my classmates, sucking the life out of people who just wanted to be friendly or helpful with my negativity.

Emotional Vampires

It took me years, but fortunately I found a therapist who helped me sort out what was underneath my behavior and alter my negative outlook. My days of being a Downer are long over.

Do I habitually seek out conflict or foment drama?

I had a chaotic childhood, and some family members chose to remain in that state for the rest of their lives. I intentionally did not.

Just because I grew up in turmoil does not mean I had to perpetuate it. I purposely spent my adulthood uncovering my destructive behavior patterns and changing them through focused attention.

I had to take a long, hard look in the mirror and reflect on my own tendencies. I saw how I was contributing to my own suffering and draining other people's goodwill. I had to accept that unappealing aspect of myself and devise an intentional plan to put myself on a path to wholeness. It was more like scratching and clawing my way to wellness.

The morning I drove my mother home from the ER, I did not feel love, relief, or even gratitude that I could be there for her. I felt only the soul-sucking experience of dealing with her own shirked responsibility yet again. There I was, as always, cleaning up her self-inflicted mess, placating her, rationalizing her behavior to other medical professionals, and stamping down my own exasperation, irritation, and inner critic, who kept reminding me, "You have to—she is your mother!"

Choosing Wellness

But that was the last time. I changed my operating system with her after that incident. Whenever she complained about her health, blamed her physicians, or tried to pull me into her emotional-vampire vortex, I mentally unhooked from her problems, changed my self-talk to "I cannot fix this," and redirected the conversation.

The day after the wedding, I kissed her good-bye, wished her safe travels on her drive home, and walked back into the house with a clear conscience and a light heart, knowing I would no longer carry the burden of her past or future choices.

Even blood, I decided, does not give anybody a free pass to suck the life out of me.

17 THE RE-POT

A repot is a metaphor on how we can break free of confinement. Repotting is about moving out of a limiting situation. When I feel stuck in what I am doing—when I am plunged into negative states of frustration, boredom, or constant fatigue—it may mean my pot is too small, my roots are bound, I need more soil, water, and sunlight. I need a bigger pot, so I have room to grow and thrive.

After four years of writing a monthly column on how federal health-policies impacted nurse practitioners, the task felt dull and uninspiring. I had loved doing it when I started; now I dreaded it.

When I find myself in uncomfortable situations, my search for the solution always starts with questions:

Why am I doing this? What is my motivation?

What makes me feel alive inside?

Is it time to quit?

Or, do I just need a repot?

Repotting does not always require changing my circumstances; I do not necessarily have to give up, quit a job, or switch careers. Sometimes my repotting happens between my ears just by shifting a mindset, considering a new perspective, or finding a more expansive context.

I knew I needed to change something about writing the column and thought about it on a vacation to France—an inspired decision. My insight did not come from the Eiffel Tower or the Mona Lisa; it came from my kindergartner's trip to a rural emergency room.

My five-year old son needed sutures after gashing his leg open on a wire at a vineyard. Within five minutes of our arrival at the ER, people swarmed to attend to him. A nurse administered nitrous oxide (laughing gas), while a physician cleaned and sutured the wound. Afterwards, the nurse handed me antiseptic cleanser, bandages, and a suture removal kit—and gave my son a courage certificate.

The whole visit took thirty minutes—and no one asked for a credit card!

When I got home, I could not wait to write my column. I contrasted my family's French emergency-room experience with American practices and fleshed out all the relevant policy issues.

Soon after at one of my son's soccer games, I noticed how his team crowded the ball, making it difficult to move it down the field. I used that as an analogy in my next column

The Re-pot

for how nurse practitioners should approach policy issues by spreading out. We need the team at the federal level – not just influencing federal bills but helping to write the regulations. We needed to be involved in state laws, local politics, and at the C-suite tables. We need to have clinically expert nurse practitioners running for office. We need more coverage.

My formerly dry and compacted root ball now started to push out new growth.

What had changed? Only my self-imposed boundaries.

The magazine's publisher never specified what I should write about, merely that the column had to address health policy. I had hemmed myself in by thinking my articles had to contain dull accounts of federal bills related to nurse-practitioner practice.

After the ER visit and the soccer game, I stopped describing dry facts. Instead, I told personal stories and used quotes and metaphors to bring policies alive. Once I let myself find inspiration anywhere, I saw it everywhere. Writing had become fun again; I even began creating original, edgy titles.

I had repotted myself. I stepped out of my routine and cleared my self-inflicted obstructions with new experiences. Sometimes it happens that way. Other times, I need to actively address my trap: take a break, seek out a larger sense of purpose, or reframe the task or a situation. We all have an unlimited number of bigger pots to grow into.

We Control Our Pots

If I had to deliver the mail, I would probably find it routine, if not outright boring. But I know one carrier who sees it as much more than putting envelopes in people's mailboxes. In his mind, he is taking care of his customers.

He stops to shoot basketballs with teenagers and encourages them to go far in life. When an elderly shut-in's mail piled up, he called the fire department to come investigate. Seeing himself as a neighborhood caretaker rather than a postal deliverer gives him a larger context for his life than his coworkers get from their daily deliveries. Not all "repots" require new external circumstances. That mailman repotted himself internally to create a sense of purpose that nourishes him.

Even if I am in a situation where I cannot swap my small space for a larger one, I can widen and diversify my internal landscapes. As Holocaust survivor Victor Frankl famously reflected in Man's Search for Meaning, "Everything can be taken from a man but one thing: the last of the human freedoms—to choose one's attitude in any given set of circumstances, to choose one's own way."

18 NEVER MEET FEELINGS WITH FACTS

We were seldom on schedule in my primary-care practice. When I saw a patient for an ingrown toenail who casually mentioned chest pain, for example, I had to immediately evaluate them for a heart attack. Their fifteen-minute appointment then ballooned to nearly an hour, which pushed back appointment times for everyone in the waiting room. Needless to say, some people became irate.

"We're backed up," our receptionist would tell them. "We have emergencies. You need to take a seat."

That kind of factual explanation only made the situation worse. The waiting patients felt their needs were being disregarded, and that no one in our office valued their time. Their irritability grew and spread throughout the room.

That kind of anger-provoking incident does not only happen in medical waiting rooms. People "lose their minds" at airline counters, standing in line at the DMV, sitting in bumper-to-bumper traffic on the highway, or any other situation when emotions hijack reason.

Emotional hijacking can happen to the most even-keeled person. When the brain receives a message of emergency or threat, its neural pathways instantly go on high alert and short-circuit reasoning. So, when I developed a clinical interest in creating more peace in our waiting room, I realized our receptionist could de-escalate that emotional hijacking if she would simply just acknowledge the patients' emotional state.

My psychiatric nursing courses had wide applications that have been useful throughout my entire life.

"Never meet a feeling with a fact," I told her. "Say something like, 'I can see how upset you are at being kept waiting and in the dark. I would be upset too. I'll go get an update for you."

Validating the other person's experience with no judgment—and definitely no facts—brings them back to themselves, makes the encounter more productive, and clears the highly charged emotional energy from the room.

Emotional Barriers

A patient who had no neurological symptoms with no indication for surgery said: "This medicine isn't working. I've been doing what you said for two weeks, and I'm not making any progress. I think I need to see a spinal surgeon for this horrible back pain."

Never Meet Feelings With Facts

In my early career, patients sometimes doubted my competence because I was not a physician. When I encountered that resistance, I addressed it through their emotions, not their physical symptoms.

I said, "I get the sense you don't trust my knowledge on treating low-back pain. Do you have some underlying fear about this?"

"I'm worried I can't exercise for the foreseeable future. Exercise really calms me down. I'm not getting better, and my anxiety is going up."

"What if you did some recumbent bike training?" I suggested. "As long it doesn't hurt your lower back, we can keep you moving while we treat the pain."

Addressing the patient's real fear (their inability to exercise) rather than its proxy (my competence) raised their emotional awareness, unearthed their underlying concern, and let me offer a remedy to move forward. Imagine if I had met their initial frustration with facts instead.

I have been treating low-back pain for twenty years and just presented an update on it at a recent professional conference. It is not our practice to send patients to a surgeon when they have no surgical indications such as leg pain or motor weakness. Your x-rays and deep tendon reflexes are all normal, and there is no incontinence.

That response might have filled in some information gaps, but it would not have helped the patient at all; it did not address their real need or offer a solution. In fact, it would probably have raised their anxiety by making them feel bad about how bad they were feeling!

Three Ways to Listen

As a nurse, I learned "therapeutic use of self." I let patients know that I hear them; that I understand their health concerns and vulnerabilities; that I will not judge them; and that I am actively curious about their experience and feelings. I do not give advice; I accompany them while identifying unmet needs. This is global, or Level Three listening.

Level Two is empathic listening, being present and paying attention, but only to the other person's words, not to what is behind those words. The listener does not consider gestures, tone, or what is not being said, so they do not make any "intuitive hits." In other words, they do not tap into their own intuition to figure out what is really going on.

I go to great lengths to avoid Level One, half, or pretend listening. People do that when they are distracted with other matters and mostly focused on how they are going to respond, not on what the other person is saying, experiencing, or feeling. Level One is the kind of listening that makes people feel unheard, uncared for, and dissatisfied.

I strive to listen at Level Three, which uses all the senses to hear what the other person says and does not say, and to notice if their gestures and tone align with their words. It allows a lot of silence and relies on intuition to acknowledge the other person's words or ask ever-deeper questions. As a result, the person feels recognized, understood, and cared for. Level Three listening lifts both me and the person I am listening to, creating a warm glow of connection between us, if only for a moment.

Level Three listening goes a long way toward calming neural pathways, defusing tirades, and building trust. Anyone, at any time, can be a "therapeutic self" to others— by simply never meeting a feeling with a fact!

19 CHOOSE WISDOM

I had just delivered a presentation to a large group of nurse practitioners on patient engagement. I felt good about my content, delivery, and interactions with the audience. As I enjoyed the after-presentation glow from a job well done, I glanced at my phone. I had over twenty text messages from friends and relatives about an offensive post on my personal social-media page. Some had even contacted the platform to take it down.

Although curious, I did not seek out the original message. Instead, I called a friend, who told me the post had come from "Mary," an estranged relative. I hung up, shocked. This was an unprovoked missile. I had not spoken to Mary in three years.

What could she be ranting about?

Part of me wanted to read the post and speculate about what might have provoked the nastiness. But that would obliterate all the joy I had just been feeling and set off a week-long ordeal of anger, blaming, and trying to find a way to forgive her.

So instead, I took a ten-second pause and asked myself: "What would a wise person do in this situation? What does a person in full command of herself do when an unexpected, unprovoked missile like this threatens to disrupt her life?"

The answer was immediate and shockingly clear: She would not read it. She would disarm or deflect it.

I had a friend enter my account and take it down.

That one question, "What would wisdom look like right now?" turned out to be a game changer for me. It was the first time I chose to not let someone's hurtful behavior land in my mind, take residence, and thrust me into the dark place I knew so well.

I never read the post. I decided it had everything to do with the author. They just used me to project their own pain—although, in the heat of the moment, I sometimes find it difficult to pause long enough to remember that truth.

Yet I did. I paused, I thought, and I chose wisdom over reactivity, a remarkable step on my journey to wellness. I learned in that one tiny action, deciding to not read the post, means that I now know I do not have to react, even to personal attacks. This is true emancipation, and once experienced it cannot be unlearned.

A Long Road

My efforts at rescuing Mary started three years before the hostile post. I had sent her a check to fill her prescriptions, and she hoarded the medication to attempt suicide. Family members planned her funeral during the eight days she spent in the Intensive Care Unit. No one thought she would pull through.

Mary's eighteen-year-old daughter, who was just three weeks into her first college semester, and high-school age son, were forced into the very adult roles of making life-and-death decisions for their mother. It was a harrowing, gut-wrenching time for all of us, but mostly for them.

When she finally pulled through, she refused all offers of love and encouragement. Nothing anyone said or did could motivate her to seek treatment for her long-standing mental illness and drug-and-alcohol abuse. "I have a million-dollar hospital bill to pay off, so I need money," she insisted.

After she was released and recovered enough to refuse help, I consciously decided to avoid her.

I really had no choice.

It was one thing to honor her free will and her right to refuse treatment, but I had learned from dealing with my sister Ellen's drug addiction to not carry responsibility for others if I did not have decision-making authority. So, I had to put down Mary's burden entirely. No more worrying, rescuing, funding, or arguing. I had to embrace estrangement—the loss of a previously existing relationship between family members, through physical and/or emotional distancing. It was the healthiest choice for me, and since Mary refused all help, it was the logical choice for her, too.

I discovered that while family estrangement seems hard, it is common. Some people cut one person out of their life; others walk away from their entire family; and still others limit their interactions to phone, email, or short, annual visits. Estrangement is a very individual choice. I cut Mary out of my life but kept up my relationship with her kids.

I used to be horrified by the idea of estrangement; after all, family is supposedly the most important thing in life. We get together for every holiday; we exchange gifts, we pop the cork, we gather for meals. What would Thanksgiving or Christmas be without family? Who would I celebrate my birthday with, if not family?

But Mary taught me estrangement is a healthy response to unsolvable, unhealthy relationships, especially when I have tried everything else. For me, it was framed as a boundary solution rather than a problem. And while I was initially afraid I would regret cutting ties with her, I ultimately felt liberated from the tragic situations she kept creating for herself, over which I had absolutely no impact or control.

Shared DNA did not require me to stay in abusive relationships or continue witnessing determined self-destruction. Whenever I start feeling the slightest bit of guilt or doubt in difficult decisions, I can remember to choose the thing that brings me the most freedom, to choose freedom over anything else.

20 PARENTING TEENS

As every parent knows, teenagers cause their own type of distress and worry. I certainly did; I started drinking when I was twelve years old and was arrested three times before I was sixteen.

It is helpful to understand the Hierarchy of Needs as defined by Abraham Maslow, the father of Humanistic Psychology, so we can grow into adults who can self-regulate and have social interest in others. We can't reach our human potential unless we have our basic needs met. Our first need is for physical safety, food, shelter and water. Then we need to feel safe and secure. Then we grow a sense of belonging, intimacy and friendships which become vital in adolescence.

Once we have a sense of belonging, we have a greater capacity to go out into the world and explore, learn and grow, take risks. Like a ship having a safe harbor, the boat first must be seaworthy before it goes out into the wild ocean. It's the exploration *along with* the safe harbor that sets up conditions for someone to become a truth-seeking, authentic, purposful, humanitarian, creative, morally intuitive, and equanimitous person—a self-actualized person—and reach their highest potential. It's the exploration *along with* the safe harbor that sets up conditions to become self-actualized and reach our highest potential.

My parents' response to their six adolescents' need to rebel against them and conform to their peer group was to yell, ground, demean, insult, withhold love, and beat.

I knew many people who reacted like my parents. First, they yelled or hit; then, after they calmed down, they came in and tried to make it all better with their child.

Sometimes, they skipped that second part.

My husband and I wanted a different approach. We did not like to yell, and we never wanted to hit our children. We wanted to live by the "Connection Always Before Correction" adage—we would connect with them before we said or did anything else, so they knew we had their back.

So, to place connection before correction, we adopted these practices learned in our parenting classes:

- *Wide Freedom.* We set clear expectations for our two sons, gave them freedom to make their own decisions, and then let them face the consequences.
- *Three Strikes.* If they got caught doing anything idiotic, destructive, impulsive, or illegal—stealing,

vandalizing, drinking, or using drugs, all things I admittedly got caught at when I was a teenager—that was Strike One.

- *Involve Kids in the Consequences.* Then the three of us would discuss and agree to a plan about what the correction should be.

If they did it again, we would use the same routine—but that would be Strike Two.

A third strike-worthy mishap between the ages of thirteen and eighteen would indicate a pattern of bad behavior, requiring drastic intervention like boarding or military school.

Thankfully, neither of our boys made it to three strikes. The oldest only got a single strike, and the youngest only got a half strike as the result of his seventeenth birthday party.

I had arranged the party as a surprise. My husband and I invited twenty of his friends, set up food and soft drinks, and then naively left the house to attend a play. Just after intermission, my cell phone vibrated. I checked it out of habit and saw that was from the police department.

I stepped outside the theater to take the call as a knot of worry started to gnaw at my gut.

"This is Eileen O'Grady," I said, trying to calm my pounding heart.

"We're at your house and need to inform you an underaged girl had been taken to the emergency room for being unresponsive. More than two dozen kids took off on foot when we got here; your son stayed. We found alcohol and marijuana all over the house. Did you provide it?"

"No officer. I left ninety minutes ago. I only supplied food and soft drinks."

"Well, you need to get home. We'll wait here with your son until you do."

Later we learned the girl's mother was the one who called for an ambulance after seeing a picture on social media of her daughter passed out at our house. Following protocol, the police showed up as well, and, finding alcohol, pot, and a pipe made from a Gatorade bottle, searched the house from top to bottom, going through every closet and looking under every bed. When we got there, two officers were sitting with him in our living room.

"Your future is over," one was telling him. "You'll never see college. We're sending the pot to the lab, and if there's anything else in it, you could be looking at jail time.

"If the kids who fled get arrested for drunk driving or hurt anybody, you and your parents will be held liable.

"And I'm gonna call your principal and let your school security know exactly what took place here," he went on.

"You might not even graduate high school."

I was confused and concerned by all these threats, but seeing the fear in my son's eyes, the very first thing I did was hug him, so he knew his father and I had his back. Connection before correction, always, is the cornerstone of the three-strike rule. Putting our relationship above all else let him know he was loved in that moment, no matter what. We would get through the rest together.

In the end, the police let him off with just a warning. When they finally left, my husband and I surveyed the house. It was a mess, littered with plastic cups, some still filled with soft drinks spiked by the oversized, nearly empty bottle of Kirkland vodka standing on the kitchen counter. The kitchen table had obviously been used for beer pong.

"What happened?" I asked. "How could you be so irresponsible?"

"I wasn't! I didn't even know about the party—you did that! I didn't invite anybody! They're the ones who brought the booze and the weed. I had nothing to do with it, and I couldn't stop them. It was me against everybody else!"

And then the three of us sat down to discuss what was going on in his young life, a conversation that could not have happened without the strong connection we already had with each other.

"Are you drinking?"

"Yeah. I drank at the party, and I have a beer now and again."

"Are you using pot?"

"Yeah, but not a lot! Just now and then. You know, with my friends."

"Are you trying to escape from something?"

"No! I'm just… trying to fit in. Go along with the crowd."

Maslow would describe this as "belonging" behavior for a teenager.

We talked about my family's history and my own alcoholism. Did he have any early signs of addiction? No, definitely not.

We explained—again—the impact alcohol and pot have on a developing brain.

"None of your friends had the courage to stay with you and shoulder some of the responsibility," we pointed out. We talked about what makes a good friend and what "having your back" looks like.

"It isn't fair," he protested angrily. "I never wanted the party! And now I'm in trouble for what other people did!"

The three of us agreed he had to clean up the mess, make sure his friends had all gotten home safely, and check on the girl in the hospital.

"Since you didn't run away and are accepting the consequences," I said, "I think this is only deserves half a strike—especially since I initiated the surprise party. I'll never do it again," I promised.

"Only half a strike?" he said. "Okay, I guess that's fair."

Despite the mess, I felt pretty good about how the situation ended. The girl was okay and was sent home. He knew we really loved him and had his back—something I never experienced in my own childhood. The three-strikes rule worked for all four of us: it gave our sons autonomy within specific parameters of how far they could push the envelope, reminded us to expect rebellion and be prepared for screw-ups, and kept us from freaking out when our kids did something wrong.

Thanks to the conscious framework we used, we could see our boys' errors in the context of their evolving adulthood. The teen years, we came to realize, are an older (and, admittedly, scarier) version of the terrible twos. Rule-breaking and acting-out are nerve-wracking but nevertheless necessary in both rebellion stages so the child can develop and gain autonomy. We can never know the full truth of a teenagers life, we can only approximate what they may be experiencing.

For the boys, the framework not only made us approachable—they knew they could come to us when they made mistakes and we would not overreact—it also gave them sanctuary and unconditional support as they struggled with the massive brain-chemistry fluctuations, unpredictable hormonal surges, and unrelenting peer-group pressure.

As a consequence, we all became closer, and I added the three-strikes rule to my arsenal of high-level wellness tools—especially the "connection before correction" concept. I use it whenever I run into situations with employees, siblings, or even friends.

I used it when I pulled that nurse out of the meeting when she was being bullied. I acknowledged her feelings before talking about how to handle situations in the future. I used it when I spoke to the physician who had done the bullying, as well. I first reminded him he was a good guy and how his outburst was out of character before we talked about making amends to the nurse.

I used it when I had made that horrible mistake of giving a nondiabetic insulin and had to approach a known bully to admit my error. I went out of my way to make a connection—understanding his concern and appropriate anger—before I addressed the fix.

I even taught it to my receptionist for those times when the waiting room was full and patient irritation was boiling over. We are, after all, all human beings, all social creatures. We need our emotions and experiences acknowledged, especially when anger or despair or fear flares up. When I go out of my way to make connection first, it replaces the me-versus-you attitude with an "us" mentality, which smooths the road and eases the pain of the correction.

21 GRIEF, GUILT, AND GROWTH

My youngest son was two when a miscarriage left me raw and wracked with grief. When I witnessed my father's death five days later, my grief engulfed me. I was overwhelmed, but my heartache was uncomplicated—as pure and uncomplicated as the love that connected us. It came with such force, it felt like childbirth. Waves of unstoppable pain gathered momentum and wracked my body. I had no influence over it. I cried for two full days, walking the deserted country roads around my parents' home in rural Connecticut. My entire psyche sobbed uncontrollably, leaving me spent as the tears and mucus poured out.

In his eulogy, I told a story to describe how good and kind he had been. When I was a teenager, a friend who was being physically and sexually abused by her father ran away to our house. My sisters and I hid her and fed her without either her parents or mine knowing.

Her father eventually showed up at our door in a rage, demanding his daughter and threatening what he would do if we did not produce her immediately.

My father quietly walked outside and asked the huge man to leave our property. He did not know all the details of her situation, but he felt the truth of the matter deep down and listened to his gut. He refused to even ask us if she was in our house; no way would he simply turn her over to this very dangerous and raging man.

I have always cherished him for that, even though it did not change the outcome. When the police came, they forced my friend to go home with her abusive father, no questions asked. But my father's courageous attempt to defend her made him a hero in my mind. I deeply admired his goodness, his gentleness and loyalty, his brave, expansive heart, and his unexpected sense of humor.

He had a number of chronic illnesses. I sat with him in the Intensive Care Unit once after he had a heart attack. Getting sleepy, I took out my contact lenses and put them in two paper cups on his bedside table.

When I woke up, the cups were gone.

"Dad, what happened to the two cups on your tray?" I asked.

"The nurse brought my pills while you were asleep," he replied. "She probably took the cups away after I washed them down. Why?"

"I think you drank my contact lenses."

"Great," he said, without missing a beat. "So now I'll be able to see out of my ass!"

Memories like those comforted me as I walked the country roads, even as they pointed to what I had lost. But not all loss is so simple.

My mother and I had a far more complex relationship. When she died two years after my father's death, I felt sadness, regret, guilt—and, admittedly, relief.

Unfortunately, I did not have the time alone as when my father passed to deal with all those conflicting emotions. My siblings and I had already gathered for her final days, so we spent that time and the days immediately afterward planning the funeral, notifying far-away family, and picking people up from airports, etc. None of us had any time to feel, much less process, our loss.

"I'll grieve when I can get back to normal life," I told myself. But unprocessed emotions do not dissipate; they stay buried. Mine remained suppressed until about a year after her funeral, when I decided to do a four-day vision quest. I had to completely disengage from my daily schedule and concerns before I could sort through the issues and unaddressed grief about my mother—not to mention Ellen, my nephew's diagnosis, my own addiction and my own miscarriage.

By then, it was long overdue. I had been fortunate to have time and space when my father died, but I did not get to choose the circumstances around all my other losses.

If I had, my fears and grief and distress would not have simmered inside for so long and erupted into such destructive and erratic behavior.

Your Blues Ain't Like Mine

Experts used to talk about Elisabeth Kubler Ross' five stages of grief, but now they acknowledge grief as highly individualized and often has no identifiable stages or process. Loss and sorrow cannot be formulaic; trying to "fit" our emotions into a pattern or feel them on schedule merely causes more pain and brings on more guilt. Yes, guilt is often a byproduct of loss. Parents can become overwhelmed with guilt when they lose a child. Spouses may feel it when they lose their partner. Sometimes people feel guilty about not having repaired a relationship or apologized for an imagined slight.

We all have or will lose our parents, and it will hit us all differently, depending on our age, our relationship, and how they die. Some people will never feel whole again. Others will eventually discover a new freedom in their loss. Still others will learn to let go and move on. Those different reactions are why most cultures and religions designate mourning periods, distinctive dress, and other rituals to alert the community about our loss and need for space to grieve.

I urge you to take that space when you experience a loss and use it to acknowledge the full force of your emotions. Go ahead and let the pain wrack your body, like the agonizing waves of childbirth. Do not try to stop the grief or "be okay;" just accept it and let it pass on its own, no matter how long it takes. Even if you are suddenly overwhelmed weeks, months, or years later by a smell, a sound, an image, or a memory, let it be part of consciously releasing guilt and choosing wellness.

I loved my parents and Ellen and still miss them, but I no longer tear up when I remember seeing them take their last breath. I used to believe the day would never come when I did not cry. But it did.

Complicated Grief

Losing my father was almost easy compared to losing my mother. Dad and I had a great relationship. He was good down to his soul, and I always knew he loved and supported me.

But my mother's passing was muddled with overlapping remorse, anger, guilt, and a huge sense of relief that caused more guilt. I probably could not have processed all those conflicting feelings even if I did have the time and space to walk country roads and cry like when my father died. My emotions for and about my mother were far too jumbled, raw, and confusing to sort though, name, and resolve without my vision quest's liberating immersion-into-self.

But as knotty as that grief was, losing someone to suicide, murder, or accident is far more complicated. It unavoidably ignites guilt, even though we had nothing to do with the death. The pain is devastating. When Robin Williams committed suicide, his best friend, Billy Crystal, said over and over, "No words."

He was beyond inconsolable. He had to find his own solace—and he could not do it in public.

When Others Grieve

I did not want anyone to try and make me feel better when I was grieving. I did not want to hear, "He's in a better place." Or, "It's all part of God's plan." Or, "At least she's not in pain anymore."

I wanted to be met where I was, not have my grief cheapened with clichés or advice or well wishes.

Do not tell a grieving person what they are feeling or going to feel. Do not tell us how to handle tomorrow or the next day.

Just acknowledge that nothing is okay.

If you can, communicate some personal truth:

"I'm so sorry to hear about your father passing last week. I can't imagine what you're going through."

"I loved your mom. I'm going to miss her, too."

"I really don't know what to say. I'm just so sorry for your loss."

When a deeply compassionate friend said, "Remember, what you're feeling is not a permanent state," I held onto it for months.

Grief, Guilt, and Growth

When we choose wellness, even loss can expand our emotional awareness. It can make us more compassionate, turn our focus toward what really matters, and, best of all, remind us how deeply we have loved.

22 THE WISDOM OF CELLS

The 2013 Nobel Prize in Physiology went to three scientists, Rothman, Schekman and Sudhof, who discovered the cell membrane, not the nucleus (i.e., the brain), is the wonderfully precise mechanism behind the cell's transport system. It was a Nobel Prize-worthy discovery that uncovered an ancient fundamental aspect of how cells shuttle cargo around. When I read that there is an intelligence to how the most basic form of human life relies on their membranes to import and export molecules, I had a flash of my own, albeit unrelated, inspiration on human boundary-setting. Why not take their truth about how our cells work and apply it to our external lives? If the tiniest cellular elements in our bodies know how to intelligently erect boundaries, can we do the same on the macro level?

The Nobel laureates determined that our cell membranes have three functions: to decide what comes in, what goes out, and what to dock to. Suppose we laser-focused on those same three functions to frame our life as we pursue wellness.

What We Let In

Our cell membranes are not only semi-permeable; they have a discernment system of their own. When they function properly, they recognize and keep out harmful substances. When they do not function properly—they get overwhelmed with toxins, for example and they mutate, which leads to cellular death.

Which eventually leads to our death.

That is the micro level, but I like to think it all starts on the macro level with the toxins and nutrients we let into our lives: The food and drinks we ingest. The people we allow into our inner circle. The books, magazines, and web content we read. The news, TV shows, and movies we watch. All the healthy-happy vs. harmful-disturbing elements we encounter every day. Too often, we allow it all to just "hit us" rather than sort through what we will and will not absorb into our minds and, by extension, our bodies.

Anything we cannot control, or damages our relationships, or affects our wellbeing is potentially toxic. I am an alcoholic, so alcohol is toxic to me—I cannot control my intake once I start. I can only abstain from drinking.

"News junkies," who cannot stop keeping one eye on the latest headline, blog, and tweet, get a twisted sense of reality from their perpetually negative diet, and their body responds to their constant outrage by continuously squirting cortisol, the fight-or-flight stress hormone, into their bloodstream. Cortisol not only affects mood and sleep, it skews conversations, alters eating habits, and, yes, stops the body from releasing extra weight.

Any activity we cannot control—be it video gaming, TV watching, shopping, eating, fixating on social-media, or porn—cuts us off from real-world interactions that provide the connections we need to flourish as human beings. Even people can drain and deplete us, as I certainly discovered before I started creating invisible protective boundaries and edited out the vampires, naysayers, bullies, know-it-alls, and even dark teachers of my life. I devised two tools to help me filter incoming toxins.

The Suburban Driveway

Some friends and family are "across the street" people, who I only wave at from a distance. I briefly greet "driveway" friends outside but do not invite them into my house. I decide when and if to welcome in "front-door" friends when they knock. And I have a tiny circle of carefully selected "back-door" friends who know they need not knock at all; they have full access to me whenever they want it.

The Suburban Driveway technique gives me full agency to choose the distance I want between me and other people. For a while, I struggled with whether assigning people to slots was too judgmental. Then I remembered how much harm I endured from having no boundaries with my family members, who all believe they are part of my tiny back-door circle. DNA does not grant automatic access to me anymore; my wellness cannot withstand those kinds of constant hits. Like my cell membranes, I now know better than to let those toxins in.

Parent the Child I Have, Not the One I Hoped For

As soon as I found out I was expecting, I fantasized about who my baby would become—thoughtful, educated, athletic, and funny. He (or she) would have his father's eyes, my nose, and our combined stamina. As a beautiful mixed-race (Indian and Irish) child, he would be off-the-chart smart, have a fiery spirit, and be fun and easy to raise.

That is every parents' dream, right? But dreams seldom align with reality, and children grow up to be who they need to be, despite our efforts to influence their every thought and action.

Applying that concept to everyone in my life meant radically accepting who they were, rather than who I expected them to be. When a friend kept refusing invitations to join me for evening events, like dinner or the theater, for example, I used to get confused and annoyed. We were close and enjoyed each other's company, so it bothered me to see her cut out a third of her life. I wanted her to enjoy everything I enjoyed, the same way I enjoyed it.

When I chose to radically accept that she did not like going out after five o'clock p.m. and invited her to lunch and daytime museum trips instead, she accepted every time. Our relationship became strong, warm, and honest, and her habits no longer confused me.

Accepting some people for who they are can be a challenge. When I run across people who only talk about themselves, for example, I have to remind myself to just ask questions and not expect them to show any interest in me or anything I might want to share. I can only take those kinds of people in small doses.

I used to have a conflict-avoidant boss. I would take office problems and conflicts to her, per protocol, but she never offered solutions or provided team leadership. I finally gave up my illusion about her abilities and aligned my expectations with the reality of who she was rather than who I wanted her to be—which gave me license to step up and become the default team leader myself.

Of course, the reverse is true, as well. I no longer confide in friends who cannot or will not respond empathically. I accept that they do not conform to who I want them to be, but that does not mean they are entitled to know my vulnerabilities!

What We Let Out

Toward the end of my parents' lives, my siblings and I pleaded with them to get their affairs in order. They had two homes in two states, 1500 miles apart, accounts all over the place, and an outdated will.

"Please," I said, "it's time to get your life organized. Let's get rid of all the extra 'stuff' sitting around and make some kind of a plan."

I do not know if they simply could not or were just unwilling to get their affairs organized. But they never did. Finally, my brother said, "They live by crisis. Let's just wait for the crisis, and all the decisions will be made for them."

He was right. I put down that burden and stopped talking to them about it or even thinking about it. Rather than be continually frustrated and worried, I radically accepted that their affairs were not something I could influence in any way, and I did not need to give their lack of planning any consideration until they both died. I "let out" those wasteful, ineffective emotions and responsibilities. Learning to drop burdens that were not mine helped me devise two tools to filter my own toxic output.

Ten-Second Pause

Releasing waste feels good. When I write an angry email, for example, as I did when I worked on my dissertation, I feel cleaned and relieved. Fortunately, my "cell membrane intellect" knows to pause for ten seconds so I do not immediately hit Send. By pausing to take responsibility for the type of energy I send out, I am forced to pay attention to my own inner life as well as the patterns of those around me. I consciously choose to not engage with anyone when stress makes me tiny-hearted, mean, and critical.

Instead, I wait until I can "Send" with generosity and respect.

Notice and Acknowledge

I acknowledge nearly everyone I come into contact with. It is a simple and beautiful tool that merely requires specifically noticing who a person is, not just what they are doing.

"I really appreciate how you used your humor to break the tension in that meeting."

"I know it's not easy to call your mother so often; she can be difficult. But it really shows me how loving and compassionate you are."

"I want you to know how brave I thought you were to speak up and ask for a raise."

Wellness Docking

When cells "dock" they bind to each other to form a stable complex, they fuse together. Like molecular membranes, I strive to be intelligent about whom I dock to. Spouses, partners, friends, family, neighbors, and co-workers have enormous influence over us; they are the "docks" that bring stability—or chaos—to our lives as we absorb their emotions and behaviors. Of course, we also have enormous influence on them, but not necessarily as much as we would like. The lead-by-example concept is a wonderful ideal, but it seldom has much effect on people we have no direct authority over.

Surrounded by people who drank and smoked, I, too, drank and smoked. When I took up running, I gathered with other runners, not with couch potatoes, and ate the kind of healthy foods they ate. Docking with like-minded others made it easier to maintain my wellbeing and thus promoted my higher self and potential.

That does not mean I confine my life to only like-minded people. A family friend always brings his own junk food when he comes to visit. No one in the house will touch it and we all still love him, but I do not "dock" with him. Instead, I set up mental boundaries and pay more attention to what I am doing. I enjoy having him in my life, but my wellness-membrane-mechanism puts me on high alert, so I do not slip back into his way of life.

Since I also cannot physically disconnect from everyone who puts me in harm's way—no one can—I set up the same kind of intelligent boundaries, or mentally disconnect, whenever I have to deal with abusive, vampire-ish, or self-destructive people.

Filtering who and what I allow into my life; consciously choosing what I put out to others; and intentionally making connections or setting up boundaries has been wonderfully emancipating—and I will never let that feeling go!

23 FROM VICTIM TO EMPOWERED

I love helping people find relief. After working for nearly two decades as a nurse practitioner, I began to feel distress about how few of my patients actually got better or became whole as a result of our relationship. As a nurse practitioner, I learned how to look at the whole person and the crucial role that their environment plays in their health. Once I got into practice, I was forced to narrow the focus to a body part or a symptom in a seven-minute office visit. So, I would quickly assess them and dispense advice; lose weight, eat more vegetables, quit smoking, exercise, over and over and over.

Each day I doled-out fistfuls of prescriptions to treat diseases resulting from their lifestyles. The things they were doing in between our visits were harming their health and I did not know how to change any of it—other than to prescribe pharmaceuticals. Over time my distress increased as it came into clear focus, I was just writing prescriptions for people who never took my advice. This model of care was not working for me, I was not having much of an impact. We nurse practitioners learn whole person care but are often hired into narrow medical model practices.

From all of this pain and distress I pivoted and built a new career.

Now I have a practice that has longer visits, and I have taken responsibility to understand my patients' root cause of self-defeating behavior and get them off prescription medications if possible. I have become skillful at recognizing where people are in the stages of change: resistance, thinking about it, preparing for it, doing it, or maintaining it. I now know that if you start to tell a person in resistance what do to, you drive them deeper into resistance, you are harming them. I do not dispense advice but ask far better questions, sometimes beautiful questions, to excavate what is true for each person.

Now if someone is in resistance and does not really want to change what they are doing, they want to vent or feel like they are doing something by working with me, I tell them, "We're not a good fit." If someone contacts me on behalf of someone else, I tell them, "Have the person call me." They rarely do. My intelligent boundaries ensure I only work with people seeking help and support for their own intentional change.

People like Peggy.

Choosing Wellness

Peggy sought me out because, despite trying numerous diets and exercise programs to lose weight, nothing worked long term. She would fall off the wagon after an upsetting event and stay off for months, undoing all the progress she made. Deciding to try a different weight-loss approach, she committed to six months of wellness coaching with me.

More than half my clients come for help in losing weight. My practice tilted towards weight loss after doing an NPR Talk of the Nation interview. The host asked me about a study that showed overweight physicians do not bring up weight issues with their overweight patients, so the patient does not get the support they need to make this enormous change. Instead, they are just treated for its consequences, like diabetes and heart disease.

Drawing on my own personal experience, I spoke compassionately about how hard it is to take off extra pounds. Weight loss is an adaptive problem that involves a complete mindset shift. It is not just about what we put in our mouths, but also what we put, or accept, in our lives.

I said, "No one should ever feel ashamed or alone on this journey. This is not easy."

By the time I got home from the studio, I had over 500 emails and phone calls from people around the country: professors, physicians, therapists, nutritionists, and even rocket scientists. I printed each email out and divided everyone by area code. Then I stayed up all night and called every single person back, starting with the East Coast and moving across the country to Hawaii. By the next morning, I had a new career.

So, I knew Peggy's problem was not what she thought it was—most problems seldom are. I sensed she had been gravely neglecting her own needs and desires. But as I feel obligated to provide some symptom relief when people show up, I started our first meeting by asking: "What's a typical day like for you?"

"I have to get up really early, about 5:30 a.m." she said, "because I have an hour's drive to work. And since I'm up, I'm usually the one who gets the children off to school. I have three: a nine-year-old, a seven-year-old, and a five-year-old."

"What kind of support do you have?"

"Not much. My husband is unemployed right now, but he stays up late trying to start a new business, so it's hard for him to get up in the morning. Anyway, by the time I get the kids fed and out the door, I don't have time to make breakfast for myself—or lunch, for that matter—so I usually grab a few granola bars to eat as I drive to work. By midmorning, I'm starving, but there's really nowhere to get food. I work kinda out in the boonies—there are no stores or restaurants around."

"So, you must be hungry all the time."

"Yeah, I'm hangry—hungry and angry. There's a small area with a fridge and a microwave in the break room, but that's it. Not even a coffee pot! Sometimes one of my co-workers will bring in muffins or donuts, or we'll have a cake to celebrate someone's birthday, but that's only every once in a while."

What I heard was that Peggy tolerated way too much; she over-gave and under-asked. But my job was not to give my opinion or guide her answers. Wellness coaching is an excavation process; people need to come to their own truth on their timeline. So, I simply said, "That sounds really difficult! It seems like you have so many unmet needs. Keep going. What's next?"

"I usually get home around seven, and I'm absolutely starving, so I start inhaling everything in sight. Mostly, I heat up whatever the kids had for dinner—pizza or mac 'n cheese. Something like that.

"It's always like an assault when I walk in the house. The dishes are piled up in the sink, the food is still sitting out waiting to be put away, the clean laundry is everywhere, unfolded. And the kids jump all over me as soon as I get through the door. They're starving for my attention at that point."

"And then what happens?"

"Well… my husband is usually just watching TV. He'll grill burgers and steaks for the family on the weekend, but during the week, between looking for a job and working on his business, he's too busy.

"I understand that… but you know, when I was looking for a job, I still found time to do the laundry, clean the house, make decent meals, get the kids bathed before bed... He doesn't do any of that."

She paused. "What does he do all day?!" she finished, with a tinge of surprise in her voice.

"I don't know... but keep going. I want to hear the rest."

"Well... I get pissed! Every night. I keep telling myself not to let it bother me, but when I walk through that door, I'm so hungry, all I can think about is food. I eat anything I can get my hands on, all night, until I feel sick, or I give up and go to bed."

I could see Peggy was heading for a crash-and-burn situation. I wanted to get her some relief, so when she stopped talking, I asked: "What do you want to see happen in your life?"

She thought for a moment. "I think I want... no, I do want to be a normal weight. I want to get rid of all this fat I've put on.

"And... I'd like to have a more normal life. I'd like my husband to support me more, to help around the house and with the kids. I'd like to have one single day of calm, of peace. Of not feeling like the weight of the world is on my shoulders—and I'm too hungry to think about it."

"May I make an observation?"

"Sure."

"I'm observing a lot of self-neglect, so I wonder if we could start close-in with the one thing you have complete control over: what you put in your mouth."

"But I don't know how to control my eating!" she protested.

"I'm guessing you don't respond to your hunger cues. You ignore them, so you drop down into such extreme hunger, you can't satiate it. You might benefit from a ten-point hunger scale as a place to start. One is famished and ten is overstuffed."

"What level should I be?"

"Aim to stay between four and six throughout the day."

"I think I spend most of my life at one. And then at night, I jump to 10. There's nothing in-between."

"Well, when we drop below two, we don't have the physical or emotional energy to control ourselves around food. After too long without eating, we then eat too quickly and our brain won't know our stomach is full until long after we put down our fork. That's what's going on everyday when you zoom from starving to overstuffed. Let's interrupt that pattern."

"Sounds like a good idea—but how do I do it?"

"I've known people who have lost 100 pounds, just by having a plan—but it requires time and effort and changing everything you're doing with food. It's really a mindset shift. Although, you might need to increase your budget so you can buy healthy foods and make your health a priority."

"What do I do?"

"Let's figure that out right now. What are your top three priorities?"

From Victim to Empowered

"Oh, my kids... my job, I guess... losing the weight. Maybe that last one should be number two, huh? After my kids."

"So how can you get real food into your body when you're hungry?"

"Well... I guess I could... plan a week's meals on the weekend, like I used to before I had my second baby. I could shop on Sundays and buy stuff to take with me every day. Hey—maybe I could hard-boil a carton of eggs so they're ready to go! And... I could get myself a thermos, set up coffee the night before, so it's always ready to take with me."

"That sounds like a good plan!"

Peggy implemented those small changes immediately. Within a few days, she had enough energy to create a new morning routine that included packing lunches for herself and her kids. She assigned herself a hunger-scale number throughout the day and kept yogurts and pre-made salads in the small fridge at work to keep herself between four and six on the hunger scale. We also discussed how drinking at least two liters of water every day would keep her hydrated, flush the toxins out of her system, and help stave off her hunger.

The midday meal helped, but it was not quite enough to sustain her until she got home, when she had already dropped down to a two. That is really common; people are hungriest when they first get home from work. So, she began packing a healthy snack to eat while driving home.

In time, she bought a single-serve espresso machine for work and stocked up on dark-chocolate squares so she could enjoy one square every afternoon with a cup of espresso. It was such a game changer for her—the sweetest thing she could do for herself.

Now when Peggy feels hungry, she eats real food but not to excess. Staying within the four-to-six range on the hunger scale keeps her from having a significant midday blood-sugar drop, which helps maintain her physical and mental energy. She created a space between hunger and her response to it.

All those small lifestyle modifications not only resulted in weight loss—they led to a cascade of other changes.

When starving and binging, Peggy did not have the energy to deal with her ongoing resentment about her husband's lack of support. Resetting her relationship with food empowered her to work on her troubled marriage.

She and her husband went to counseling.

Nothing changed.

She filed for divorce.

Then she fired her boss.

Out of the blue one day, Peggy mentioned that no matter how well she did her job, it was never enough for him. He expected his staff to work long hours without additional compensation, berated them for not meeting impossible deadlines, and refused to hire more help, a scenario I have heard countless times.

From Victim to Empowered

"Enough is enough," she said, and found herself a new job closer to home with far better working conditions.

But she still was not done. She reconnected with an old friend and together, they started working out in the friend's basement and taking long walks. That was huge—she was not only exercising, she was rejoining the world, expanding her life beyond just work and family.

Now seventy-pounds lighter and single, Peggy feels like a new person. She loves her new job, has started dating, and has set new standards for what she will and will not tolerate from others.

And she did all of it on her own. I merely gave her some tools and Level Three listening, so she could hear herself talk about who she was, what she was dealing with, and what her truth was. I served as her accountability partner and support system in the beginning, but she soon became her own centrifugal force. She prioritized herself, asked others for what she needed, and when they could not (or would not) comply, she left.

As a nurse practitioner, I could never have witnessed this kind of remarkable transformation; all I could do was dispense advice in fifteen-minute clinic-visit increments. As a wellness coach, I get to ask open questions and really listen—Level Three, global listening.

I felt fortunate to witness and support Peggy's growth as she stopped tolerating nonsense and took agency over her life. What an empowering experience for both of us!

24 SELF-AUTHOR THE FUTURE

Wellness coaching is never boring. There are as many roadblocks and stories as there are people on the planet. Rick, a young man in his twenties, for example, wanted to lose fifty pounds.

"Why do you want to lose weight?" I asked during our first conversation.

After hemming and hawing for a few minutes, he finally admitted, "I want a girlfriend! I'll be more attractive if I get rid of all this extra weight."

I immediately knew Rick had what he needed to overcome the obstacles to long-term change. He had linked two powerful, deeply personal motivators—to be loved and have sex—to his desire.

That was key.

"How will your life be different a year from now if you are fifty pounds lighter?"

Again, he took a moment to consider his answer. "I won't have this gut, for one thing. I'll have a girlfriend. I'll like myself more... and I'll have more confidence!"

"What else?"

"Well, hmmm... I'll eat healthy food and exercise, so my counseling clients will see me as a role model for embodying a healthy lifestyle. I'll have more energy to help them because I won't constantly be distracted by my weight and its impact on my love life."

Rick had the right idea. Visualizing his desired positive future rather than accepting his current negative state as his only choice let his brain "see" that positive existence not only as attainable, but likely. He essentially programmed himself for the better life he wanted by expecting it to be real.

Anyone can use that technique. Focusing on how awful our life is merely perpetuates our despair because our brain sees it as fixed, unalterable. Visualizing and describing a better pattern creates a compelling destination to make the changes necessary to achieve that reality.

The human brain can only achieve what it imagines; it cannot achieve what it cannot imagine.

I tell my clients to project any increment they want: one year in the future, five years in the future, or even a self-composed obituary. It can be pure fantasy. The point is to create a compass reminding the author of their ability to self-edit their story at any time.

To say "no" to anything that does not take them toward their vision. Here is mine:

Eileen died peacefully in her sleep at age 100, surrounded by her loved ones. A Nurse Practitioner who chose to shift her mission from the established medical model of health care to those seeking to take command of their health, she will be remembered for her life's work to unleash the power of human caring.

Her dedication to elevate the science and practice of nursing, help people feel understood and whole, improve healthcare, and recognize each person's unique value and response to illness was unsurpassed.

She applied a "wild creativity" to help people clarify their most cherished values to find deeper meaning in their lives. She approached every symptom as the body's cry for attention and is widely credited with dismantling the old-school, physician-only healthcare system still prevalent at the turn of the twenty-first century. Through her unique wellness practice and school, she helped thousands transcend their toxic lifestyles and health issues.

Eileen will be remembered as a deeply soulful person who stayed true to herself in all situations. Her level of physical fitness, mental acuity, energy, and lust for life defied her age up to the end.

Her sons, both self-actualized individuals, describe their mother as someone who moved gracefully through every obstacle, continuing to learn even in her last days.

Her husband of sixty-nine years stated, "Her mere presence made everything more beautiful."

I tear up every time I read that fantasy-fiction piece. Writing it truly helped me align my life actions with my projected future. Although I wrote it years ago, I have not changed one word—and I see tiny shimmerings of it starting to come true.

Tiny Steps

Rick did not use the obituary technique, but since he knew why he wanted to lose weight and could visualize a slimmer version of himself, he and I enlisted his brain in the difficult battle of the bulge.

He chain-drank soda every day, not because he loved it but simply because it was a leftover habit from childhood— yet it amounted to hundreds of empty calories and caused wild blood-sugar swings.

"I can give up the sugar-laden drinks," he said, "but I don't want to lose the carbonation." He switched to seltzer, a tiny step that scored his first lifestyle-change victory.

Rick also ate a lot of processed foods because they were easy to grab and eat. He decided to only shop the grocery store edges, where he could fill his cart with proteins and produce. That second tiny step helped him avoid buying junk food and prepackaged "food-like" substances.

His next tiny step, to read labels on everything he needed from the middle aisles, made him realize how many so-called "natural" and "healthy" products were, in fact, chemical-laden and filled with sugar disguised as high-fructose corn syrup (which the body can neither identify nor process), cane juice, and beet sugar.

Despite taking it slow and backsliding a number of times, Rick eventually learned to cook simple meals—a skill he could use to impress his projected-future girlfriend.

"I think I'm ready to start exercising," he said, after six weeks and fifteen pounds gone.

"What activities do you like?"

"Not sure," he replied. "I never played sports as a kid, and I don't do any kind of exercise. I don't really like physical stuff," he confessed.

The more we talked, the more I realized exercise intimidated him. Not only would Rick never be one of the jocks, he was afraid to even try competing with them.

"I don't think I could ever do intense running or weight-lifting," he admitted.

"Well, can I challenge you to walk around the block twice this week?"

"I'm not sure. I don't even know if I have workout clothes."

"Okay. How can you find out?"

"Well, I know I have sweatpants somewhere, and I have regular shoes. I'll have to look through my stuff to see if I have sneakers."

"What's the first step then?"

He laughed. "Take inventory of my closet! That I can do!"

Every tiny step—even as small as searching through his closet—helped Rick feel better, which made him want to keep going. Success begets success.

As it turned out, Rick did indeed have workout clothes—and sneakers. Check!

Donning them, he walked around the block once. Check!

The next day, he did it again. Check, check! Every tiny achievement nourished him; by the third week, he was walking around a nearby lake. The movement gave his body more energy and made his mood more upbeat, which increased his enthusiasm—as did the distances he walked. Within a month, that loop around the lake had evolved into a daily two-mile walk.

And then he began to run.

He soon fused his new exercise interest with his lifelong music passion. Choosing just the right tunes for his playlist stoked his motivation and added an intellectual element to his daily run. The rhythms pulled him forward, into, and through his runs, he was now fully engaged in that wellness pursuit.

When a coworker noticed Rick's slimmer, fitter body, the two of them struck up a conversation about running and eventually agreed to meet up on Sundays. That tiny step turned what had begun as a chore into a fun way to connect with other people. They soon signed up for local races, leading them to join a running community.

Six months after our initial conversation and fifty pounds lighter, Rick participated in a 5K run as part of his college-reunion weekend. He was amazed that he kept pace with the same jocks who used to intimidate him.

A few years later, he beat his own time goal in the Boston marathon. He was happier than he had ever been—except for when he went on a date with a woman who became his long-term girlfriend.

25 PULLING ROOTS VS WEED-WHACKING

"Annette, why is now the time to start an exercise regimen?"

The obese woman on my computer screen threw up her hands. "I don't have any choice! My physician says I have to lose 100 pounds, or I'll be dead in five years, and the only way I can do that is by exercising! But I hate it—I hate running, I hate lifting weights, I hate going to the gym. I'm too big. I don't fit on any of the equipment, and everybody snickers at me."

Annette's problem had nothing to do with not wanting to exercise; that was just an idea she was stuck on. Most of us would much rather blame something simple than actually examine the root of our problems; it is a lot easier and less painful. I had gotten stuck on the idea that I was depressed. I wanted to attribute all my problems to a mood disorder when the real root was alcoholism.

I did not know yet what Annette's root problems were, but I knew it was not an aversion to exercise, so I said, "Tell me more about how you got here."

"Because I don't exercise."

Feeling stuck is the common thread in why people contact me. It comes in two flavors: the diffuse, "I'm a mess" version, when the person cannot name their most pressing problem because they are too overcommitted, stressed, or overwhelmed to think clearly; and the more specific, "I need to / I hate / I can't / I'm afraid of" variety.

Annette was stuck in a specific fused thought with brought forth a false equivalency. Her idea, "I need to exercise" was fused to, "In order to lose weight." Noticing this false equivalency prompted me to ask, "Can you think of any other reason why your weight is out of control for you?"

"Well, the two liters of soda every day probably don't help, but I need those because otherwise I can't stay alert. My work is very demanding."

"Okay. Can you give me a typical day of your eating?"

"Lemme see… take yesterday. I was late getting out of the house because I kept hitting the snooze button, so I stopped and grabbed a coffee and a donut. Then… I had a few more 'cause someone brought in a fresh box of Krispy Kremes®. At lunch, I had a combo meal at Arby's. I got a candy bar from the vending machine around 2:30—you know, everybody gets kind of draggy around then, right?

Pulling Roots vs Weed-Whacking

But it was a really long, tough day. I knew I'd be too tired to cook when I got home, so I picked up some lo mein on the way and ate it with a few leftover chicken wings. Oh—and I had the leftover celery sticks that came with the wings, so at least that's a veggie, right?"

I agreed. "Right. What else?"

"Yeah. Well... I had some kettle corn while I watched TV, and a cup of hot chocolate to help me sleep."

"Can I make an observation?"

"Sure."

"Maybe it would be better if we focus on your eating habits first before we tackle exercise. I wonder if you even know when you are hungry throughout the day."

"Okay... but how do I lose 100 pounds without exercising?"

"You can't out-exercise your diet; it's too nutrient-poor. We can we start with where you are now and explore your relationship with food. We can address the root issues of your weight challenge. I think once you've successfully lost some weight, you'll feel more comfortable about moving."

"So, I don't have to feel bad about not exercising right now?"

"That's right—you don't have to feel bad about not exercising right now."

Feeling stuck is like an invasive weed. Its above-ground stem, leaves, and buds are the obvious things we want to change. But they are only manifestations of the real problem.

The weed itself runs underground with many strong roots. Those are the real problems behind our stuck-ness, and they are often false beliefs or false equals.

I, too, had sought out a therapist hoping she would solve my problem, which I falsely believed was depression. I could not seem to shake it off. I even thought I might be bipolar. Just as Annette wanted her problem to be lack of exercise, not her diet, I wanted my root problem to be anything but alcoholism.

My first therapist went along with my delusion! She dismissed my drinking as a problem, told me to cut down to one glass per evening, and assured me she could cure my depression if I just kept seeing her. So I did, until that morning in my kitchen, when I realized she had just been whacking at my weeds.

If we only cut down to the soil, we never address the root of our problems. Annette's weed looked like exercise to her, but its roots were her false beliefs about food. We examined her lifestyle to unravel those false beliefs; "I need soda to stay alert, I don't have time to plan and cook meals, I have to eat whatever is available, and, I can never refuse 'free' food."

I asked her, "Are each of those ideas opinion or fact?"

"Well, my parents drilled it into us," she replied. "They grew up poor, so they had a thing about wasting food. We kids had to eat everything, whether we liked it or not. And whenever there was free food—you know, potlucks, school functions, church coffee hours, things like that—we were told to chow down, so they didn't have to feed us whatever the next meal was supposed to be.

"What gets to me is they were doing okay moneywise by the time we kids came along, but they still acted dirt poor. I guess they were just used to operating that way. Anyway, it never occurred to me I had adopted their way of thinking about food."

Her parents' attitude about food was a powerful hidden root for Annette's obesity weed, and a good demonstration of how we cling to belief systems even when they do not serve us anymore. The parents never let go of the world view about food they learned during their early, formative years, even though that view stopped being valid when they grew up. They clung to it so strongly they handed it down to Annette and her siblings during their early, formative years.

Of course, once we see the truth about our false beliefs, we can quickly pull those weeds out by their roots. But letting go of an idea held since childhood is extremely difficult; we unthinkingly hold it as fact, which is why the eight-billion-dollar weight-loss industry keeps coming up with new simple-solution gimmicks to keep people distracted from exploring their truths. But diets only lop off the top of the obesity weed, which actually strengthens and expands its root system.

As Annette dug out her false beliefs, she learned to eat in response to hunger, not food availability, and her weight began falling away naturally. So, we kept exploring. We discovered she also used food to feel better; specifically, she ate to soothe resentment.

"I do hold grudges," she admitted. "I get angry, and then the anger turns to resentment, and then it just sticks. It never occurred to me that forgiving someone or just... not holding a grudge against them anymore would help me lose weight!"

Annette began to mindfully note whenever she became excessively aggrieved, so she could make a conscious decision about how to handle each event as it occurred. The more she deliberately looked at her reactions, the more she was able to shake off her anger and bitterness over minor incidents.

Her emotional eating diminished, more pounds dropped away, and she discovered she felt not only physically but mentally lighter. "I guess I've really been weighing myself down with my own attitude!"

Each time we uncovered another root cause for her false beliefs about food, we developed a new plan to give her more control over her eating. One day, after Annette had lost about thirty pounds, she decided to take a walk to burn off her extra energy.

Soon, she was walking a little farther every day. Losing even more weight. Feeling good about her body and her life. And exercising organically.

Pulling Roots vs Weed-Whacking

Kill Those Roots

Sometimes, we not only have to rip our weed's roots out of the ground, we have to make sure a stray tendril does not take root somewhere else.

Katie had been overweight her entire life. Despite trying countless diets, remedies, pills, patches, detoxes, cleanses, fasts, and eating plans—none of which she could stick to long term—she had never once enjoyed a single successful weight-loss experience. Her false beliefs were: "I've been obese too long to lose weight," and "Obesity runs in my family; there's nothing I can do about it." But when her fifty-something father died from complications of obesity and diabetes, she got frightened about her future.

I understood. I could not see my pathway to change until I, too, located a powerful "why": I did not want to raise my kids in the same kind of alcoholic home I had grown up in.

Katie's motivating "why" was even more powerful: her own mortality.

"What do you think is causing your overweight condition?" I asked.

"I suppose it's my sweet tooth," she said, laughing. "I'm definitely a sugar junkie."

She went on to describe binging on sugar-laden packaged food and candy. "You know," she admitted, "sometimes I don't realize how much I've eaten until I've finished the entire box of cookies. Or two. Or three," she finished, dropping her eyes. "It's like, once I start, I just don't want to stop. It can be anything: cookies, cake, cheesecake, candy. I'll eat a whole family-sized bag of M&Ms in a single sitting. I'll be terribly ashamed of myself the next morning, of course. But even so, I'll do it again that same evening."

"Are you hungry when you start one of these binges?"

She shrugged. "I don't know. Maybe. Maybe not."

"Do you ever do it when others are around?"

"No, only when I'm alone. It'd be too embarrassing if anyone saw me eat like that. Besides, when I'm alone, I don't even think about what I'm putting into my mouth.

"I just… eat."

"Let's try something. Set yourself a limit—any limit. If you can't stick to it, you may have an addiction."

Katie flunked that test, just as I had with alcohol. Realizing she was, indeed, addicted to sugar led her to finally acknowledge what she had known deep inside for a long, long time: she could not have "just one" of anything sweet. It was a life-changing moment.

Making the intentional decision to abstain from sugar, she purged it from her kitchen and set about planning meals and bringing real food into her house. She even took an online nutrition course and changed everything about how her family ate.

Nine months later, she had lost seventy pounds. She still had forty pounds to go when she plateaued. Then, ever so slowly, she began gaining weight again—the typical dieter's nightmare. "What's going on?" I asked. "What's changed?"

"I don't know!" she wailed. "I don't have any sugar in my house, I swear. No sugar."

"You've had a problem eating without thinking before. Could you be doing something like that again?"

"No," she answered, too quickly. Then she shrugged. "I'm going through some rough times, and I... maybe... I snack a little at night to feel better."

"Tell me more."

"It's... Girl Scout Cookies."

Katie had reactivated her sugar addiction, this time to soothe herself. I sensed she had yet another emotional root holding her down and making her immune to change.

"What do you want, really want?" I asked her. "Sometimes people are good with what they've achieved—sometimes, dropping a goal can be as important as pursuing one."

Katie shook her head firmly. "I want a lean body. I want to be forty pounds lighter."

"And so you're actively sabotaging that goal because...?"

"I don't know! It's very distressing!"

"Let's look at it from another angle. Since right now you cannot be committed to your success, what could you be committed to instead?"

"Committed to? You mean, like, am I committed to... failure...? No! To using food to numb my feelings?" She drew a breath. "I think so. I'm also committed to... to..."

She looked down. "I'm committed to not getting noticed."

I nodded. "Say more."

"Ever since I've been losing weight, people... look at me... and... and talk about my... my body. They check me out from head to toe like I'm some sort of... thing! And it makes my skin crawl! I've always been invisible; I never realized how invisible I really was. Their leering is so awful—OMG! Is that what's going on?" Her eyes flashed. "Is all this attention making me backpedal?! No! I will not let unwanted attention prevent me from going where I want to go! I will have the good life I want, the body I've worked for!"

"Katie, you've just connected two ideas you had never put together before: if you achieve your goals, you'll have to deal with people noticing the new you, even staring at your new body. That's a huge adjustment.

"Are you ready to take on the discomfort of people scrutinizing you?"

"Yes, absolutely!" she said emphatically.

Since Katie was more committed to achieving her weight-loss goal than to being invisible, we worked on acceptance. No, she could not control anyone else's reactions, but she could control her own. She could grow a thicker skin around body attention.

She lost those last forty pounds and replaced her previous false beliefs with three truths about weight loss:

Pulling Roots vs Weed-Whacking

1. Dieting does not work. Dieting is a temporary solution to a long-term problem. Diets, especially extreme ones that restrict calories or even real food, often achieve fast results, but are not sustainable. We get trapped into thinking a drastic measure fixes us, then so often result in more weight gain after the temporary diet. I get asked often about tips, tricks and hacks to lose weight, yet the only solution is to make permanent lifestyle changes that can be sustained over a lifetime. There is no going off.

2. Successful long-term weight loss is rarely about the food itself, but about having a healthy relationship to it. Everything hinges on this.

3. Addictions are all or nothing: we cannot just cut down or moderate our compulsions. One must first know if an addiction is present and if we continue to allow the substance to hijack us, we will enter a spiral of caving to compulsions, repenting and repeating. We must change our behavior—and that means first changing our long-held beliefs.

26 CONSIDER MASLOW

Steve had a different set of false beliefs. He did not know how to say "no."

"The more I do," he explained in our first meeting, "the more people expect from me. I became a professor so I could have an impact, you know? I wanted my research to shape international health policy. Instead, I blow my days on teaching and administrative work. I can barely stay up to date with what's happening in my own field. I mean—I haven't published a paper in over a year! I can't figure out how to get off this hamster wheel or get people to leave me alone long enough to get some work done."

His story was disturbingly familiar. During my academic career, I was expected to bring in grant money, publish research, sit on a seemingly endless number of university committees, and, of course, be an excellent clinician and teacher.

I hear the same complaint in my coaching practice all the time, no matter what industry my clients work in. In today's high-stress, high-speed environment, everyone is expected to do and produce more with less resources and help.

"You definitely sound exhausted," I said. "What's the hardest part of what you do?"

"I don't feel my life is my own. It's not what I want. I'm just pulled in so many directions."

Steve did not realize he had a choice about the pulling. He was stuck in a developmental growth stage: people-pleasing.

Adult Development

Maslow describes the developmental stages of life as a path towards transcendence- that we cannot become selfless unless and until our basic needs are met. Once our basic needs are met, the fully developed and fortunate human being resembles the best in humanity. Once we move out of deprivation, we can grow, and explore unity and harmony with oneself and the world. Contrary to what many us learned, Maslow never imagined a hierarchy that we climb and once we pass one level we never return to it again. Getting ones needs met is not a video game in which you get to one level and check the box, but rather a continuous cycling as our needs change and evolve. It is ongoing and can be simultaneous. Food, water and shelter are so primal and physical, it is easy to see how growth get stunted when these needs are not met.

Since Adverse Childhood Events (ACEs) often thwart those basic needs, and the lack of safety belonging and self-esteem thwart characteristics of self-actualization, such as truth-seeking, acceptance and purpose. That is why people with high ACE scores may have trouble moving past their deficiencies and face more barriers to growth.

But even people who had secure, loving childhoods and strong attachments—who grew out of their self-centered-ness and moved on to conformity, where their self-esteem developed with accomplishment and independence—often get stuck seeing themselves through the lens of how other people see them.

Like Steve, most people stay stuck right there. Only about two percent of the adult population ever reach self-actual-ization, their full potential—and that never happens before mid-life. This is very difficult and rare because it means one has to consistently have all of their physical needs met, must be open to making themselves psychologically vulnerable, be willing to accept the painful aspects of themselves, and be continually striving for growth and wisdom.

So, Steve, like most of the people in his world, still sought approval, love, and respect from everyone but himself. He did not realize his inability to say "no" came from needing people to like him.

Mid-Life Crisis

The transition from approval-seeking to self-authorship is a type of midlife crisis, a slow molting of the long-held beliefs that hardened into our identity like a shell. Leaving that comfort and familiarity behind means looking at the world, and our place in that world, in a new way. The critics in our head (not to mention the ones in our life) keep trying to pull us back to the status quo whenever we make a choice or take a stance outside what they feel is normal and comfortable—for them. We feel exposed, doubtful, and unanchored. Most people do not make it through those barriers.

I had to become sober to jump my hurdles. Once I stopped drinking, I found the strength and wherewithal to also walk away from my burgeoning academic career. I began authoring a new life that few people understood. I experienced the painful rawness of learning how to disappoint others.

Releasing my old perceptions of who I was and whose opinion about me were actually important was a huge shift—It required me standing in a very uncomfortable, vulnerable place. But eventually, like others who pursue growth, I transitioned, I felt more in sync with my true self when I learned to say "yes" to the right things and "no" to the requests that did not serve me—even if I was good at something or could do it easily.

Choosing Wellness

When I recognized Steve was standing on the same precipice, I told him, "Let's start with 'yes' and 'no.' What makes you fully alive? What do you want to be doing with your time? What do you want to leave on this planet as your legacy?"

"That's easy! I want to work on international-health research grants and take students on missions."

"So, that's your 'yes.' Anything that pertains to your research grants and student missions is a yes. Now, what's getting in the way of that?"

"I'm on the admissions committee, the sexual-harassment committee, and the curriculum-rewrite committee… and I say yes to all my grad students who want me on their dissertation committees."

"What's your motivation for doing all that?"

Steve took a long breath, then started and stopped a few times before admitting, "I'm really good at it. Who else is going to do it? Besides, people ask, and I don't want to disappoint them."

"Perhaps you want approval from too many people. Can I challenge you to create a list of five people who really matter to you? They do not have to be people you interact with regularly. They could be a colleague or mentor you haven't seen in years. In fact, they don't even have to be alive. Can you give it some thought and create that list?"

"I can do that right now!" Steve said excitedly. He immediately wrote up his list and put it in his wallet.

"That's your 'pre-approved approval list,'" I told him. "They're your personal board of directors—the only people whose approval matters. No one else's opinion counts."

"Okay!"

"So, the next time you're asked to sit on a committee, teach an extra class, or chair the department, give the answer that lines up with your priorities—'no'—so you can stay focused on your big 'yes' to the things that do align with your own wants and needs."

"But… what if I still worry about the other person?"

"Mentally run the decision by your pre-approved approval list. Remind yourself that person's opinion doesn't matter if they're not on your list. No one gets to dictate how we spend our time and energy just because they ask for it." I then challenged him to disappoint three people over the next two weeks and he accepted.

Steve's results were dramatic and emancipatory. Centering all his "yeses" around his research, grants, and student missions, he developed the mental muscle to disappoint people without resentment or guilt. He became a self-authored adult who no longer needed to rescue or please everyone else to feel good about himself.

The Answer to Overwhelm

I had chased external validation on the same hamster wheel Steve was on starting in my twenties when I put myself through nursing school by working double shifts as a float RN. After working sixteen hours straight, I was so bone-tired I could not tell what I needed more—sleep, food, or fluids. But, determined to take my nursing career to the next level, I did not listen to my fatigue. I powered through it to achieve my goal and make ends meet.

That short-term necessity developed into a long-term habit when I decided to pursue one master's degree after another, all the while being a nurse practitioner in an outpatient clinic three days a week, teaching another two days, and grinding through sixteen-hour shifts as a weekend float nurse. I remember little about my life that decade other than work, study, repeat.

Like Steve, I created my own overwhelm.

I became nauseated on the flight home from my honeymoon in Spain—just in time to start my doctoral program which had started while I was away.

Though my discomfort continued for days, I did not have time or even know how to listen to what my body was trying to tell me. I plowed ahead with the PhD program, even when I developed a full-on migraine, complete with aura and vomiting. It was the first and only migraine I ever had.

My heart was not in it—I just wanted to capture the degree—but I was too busy and exhausted to realize that. And since I had spent years ignoring my physical, emotional, and psychological needs, I did not notice when my weariness deepened into a different kind of stress.

Consider Maslow

I could not relax; I could not even sit still. I always had to be in motion. I did not know how to turn off my frenetic pace. School had become a series of meaningless hoops to jump through and not instructive. Like Steve, I was no longer aligned with my own priorities.

A planned pregnancy after four years in the PhD program gave me a strong motivation to change my life. I did not want our infant to be exposed to a tightly wound, highly stressed mother.

I had stumbled into adulthood with a core sense of unworthiness, needing repeated external validation to achieve self-esteem. Adding letters after my name was supposed to convince me that I mattered, that I was okay and worthy, but being pregnant made me realize I wanted more out of life. I felt a primal pull to reclaim my body, my relationship with my husband, and the friendships I had let fall by the wayside. I needed free time back in my life.

So, I gave up my clinical practice and weekend RN position and kept only my part-time faculty role and full-time grad student obligations. I scheduled outings with friends and visited others who lived outside my community. I made time to hike in old forests, go for regular massages, and do whatever else called to me. With the energy born of spaciousness and time to rest, I gradually gained a peacefulness I had never before allowed myself to feel.

I began the slow process of growing into a more centered, grounded individual. It was not a switch, but a slow molting, a seed that brought forth a change in mindset. Once I experienced this growth and a better way to approach life, it could not be un-learned—and my patients and loved ones reaped the benefits of my new generosity, thoughtfulness, and presence.

27 STUCK IN OLD PATTERNS

I can often personally relate to my clients' problems, but when Ron sought my help to overcome his self-diagnosed panic attacks, I had no pre-existing framework to fall back on, no preconceptions about the roots of that symptom.

"Tell me what's going on," I prompted at our first session.

"Well," he said, "I get really anxious starting about noon every Sunday. I can't relax or even calm down. I used to run when I got anxious, but these days I'm so worn down and tired I just flop on the couch with a beer and watch whatever game is on—even if it's basketball. I hate basketball! The more I stare at the TV, the more anxious I get; the more anxious I get, the more beer I drink, until I talk myself into walking into my boss's office the next morning and quitting on the spot! But I never do. I'm a mess. And a coward. It's no wonder I keep having panic attacks!"

"Okay… tell me about your work."

Choosing Wellness

"I love my work. I do. And I'm good at it. My annual reviews are always good. Excellent, in fact, and my bonuses are bigger than everyone else's. I know; I've checked. My company sets up community and civic responses to climate-change dangers. That's important to me, 'cause I'm an outdoor kind of guy."

"Then, why do you want to quit?"

"It's my boss! He sets these impossible demands. He's there before six a.m. every day and never leaves until, like seven! And I have to match him hour-for-hour—he's made that clear—or I'll lose my job, like the guy before me. But even if I get up at four-thirty a.m., he's already there! The guy is relentless! When am I supposed to get in a run? If I don't run in the morning, I lose focus later in the afternoon—and I still have hours to go just to keep up with him!"

"Tell me more."

"I want to quit so bad—I can't stand these panic attacks! I used to go camping every weekend—I need to be outdoors, okay? I need to be in nature —but I can't pull it off anymore. He's killing me! He can be a workaholic all he wants, but that's so not me! I'm no Type A, have-to-work-every-min-ute-of-every-hour-of-every-day kind of guy.

"I mean, I love my job, don't get me wrong—I just hate working for that guy. I hate him. His pushing, pushing, pushing is making me physically ill.

"I wish I had the courage to quit. I just don't wanna give up the job."

Stuck in Old Patterns

"Okay," I said when he finally ran down. "Suppose you could wave a magic wand to create the ideal situation. What would you do?"

Ron grunted. "I'd have the same job with normal hours. I'd go back to running every morning, and hanging out with my friends on Friday nights, and camping on the weekend."

"What's getting in the way of that?"

"I told you! My boss! If I don't keep up with him, he'll make my life at work miserable—or fire me!"

"Job loss is a reasonable fear," I acknowledged. "But... is it possible your boss doesn't expect you to work the same hours he works?"

"He does!"

"How do you know? Has he told you that?"

"No, but ... he makes it clear."

"What does he do to make it clear?"

"He ... he's always there, always working!"

Trapped in a generalized and toxic thought loop, Ron deflected all responsibility for his stuckness.

I asked, "Is it possible you could be wrong? Could it be that your boss just likes to work?"

"Anything is possible—but I doubt it. He's made his expectations pretty clear."

"How can you find out for sure?"

"I have no idea."

Ron's false beliefs were so deeply rooted at this point he did not even realize he was in resistance.

So I tried another angle. "Okay. Well, are there any other measures that point to whether or not you're doing a good job?"

"Yeah, I told you," Ron said. "My annual reviews are always good. My bonuses are always good."

"So, you meet those standards?"

"I more than meet them! I'm always the top performer. But he never acknowledges that—he only ever talks to me about problems."

"Does that experience or feeling seem familiar to you?"

"No!" Ron insisted. "Well, kinda. Yeah. My dad. He didn't push me like this, but nothing I did was ever good enough. He left me 'big footprints' to fill. That's what he'd say all the time. He was a quarterback. I was only full back. He pitched on the varsity team; I only played first base—but I won Most Valuable Player two years in a row! I even came close to being picked up by the minors, but you know what he said? 'How're you gonna make a living when you can't play anymore?' So, I gave it up. I mean, he obviously didn't think I was good enough to go the distance."

Ron had just uncovered the roots of his Sunday anxiety. He was not having panic attacks about work. He was experiencing generalized anxiety from repeating an old pattern—wearing himself out trying to please someone who never expressed approval. He was ignoring his body's cues and just plowing through, but he needed an immutable story to hang his helplessness on.

Just like when I had chased all my degrees.

As a wellness coach, I do not dictate advice to my clients as an authoritative expert. I know they must solve heir own problems, which, most of the time, requires a mindset change. So, every time Ron said he "just knew" what his boss expected from him, I asked, "How can you find out for sure?"

It took some time, but Ron finally blurted, "Okay, fine! I'll talk to him! But don't blame me when it gets me fired!"

He did not get fired—he got surprised. It turned out his boss had only started putting in long hours after his wife died as a way of avoiding the home they had lived in together for over forty years. By the time Ron joined the company, the man was so used to doing twelve-hour days, he no longer thought about it. But he never expected anyone else to work the same hours. He had "naturally assumed" Ron had his own reasons to come in early and stay late. He also assumed Ron's consistently high annual-review ratings and bonuses adequately communicated his approval, since he was "not much of a talker."

All of Ron's false beliefs got uprooted in that one conversation. "I shoulda sat down with him sooner," Ron admitted. "He's really an okay guy. He just doesn't like to talk a lot."

Once he realized his own emotional pattern, Ron mindfully weaned himself from unquestioned approval-seeking. He went back to running every morning, which not only relieved his anxiety, but sent him to the office in a good mood every day. Eventually, he even realized he enjoyed working long hours, although not as many as his boss did. He learned to consciously decide when it was time to knock off and go home every day.

He was finally free and in the land of choice.

28 POLARITY PROBLEMS

Ruth did not have a false-narrative problem like Ron. Instead, she had a conundrum that needed to be leveraged, a point of tension that needed to be managed.

"Tell me what's going on," I said in our first session.

"I love my work, and I love my children—but I enjoy the office more than spending time with my elementary-school-age kids, and I'm overwhelmed by guilt about it. I feel bad all the time."

A mother and a lawyer, Ruth had a not-uncommon family-career polarity. Unlike my alcohol addiction that required one side to completely vanquish the other, her perpetual tension was like inhaling and exhaling—both equally important. She could not resolve the issue by choosing one part of her life over another. She had to find a way to leverage both of them. When we charted her weekly schedule, she discovered how much she allowed her work to seep into nearly every aspect of her life.

"I'm a partner in my firm. I get paid very well to bring in big accounts and resolve client issues. At work, I feel competent—I know what I'm doing—and I get recognized.

"At home… that's a completely different story. The house is always in chaos—the noise, the mess, the constant demands and needs for attention. As soon as I figure out one child's problem, another kid pops up with a different one—all while I'm trying to handle work texts and emails, prepare meals, or chauffeur them here and there between phone calls."

"What is your parenting style?"

"Parenting style?! Uh… Okay, I know I'm too permissive, and the kids get away with a lot that other mothers wouldn't allow. But they take advantage of me, so sometimes I blow my top! Then I become an Army general, and I hate being pushed and pulled like that. Why can't they understand?"

"I can see the upsides of being at work," I said. "What are the upsides of being home?"

"I love my kids."

"What else?"

"Well… hmm. There aren't any, really. No one enjoys it when we're all together. Probably because I'm so… volatile."

"So, what does work? What do you enjoy?"

"I'm not sure." Ruth paused. "We all like apple picking, ice skating, visiting county fairs, that kind of thing. I usually leave my phone at home when we go on those kinds of outings. But we only do that stuff a few times a year."

Polarity Problems

"What kind of mother do you want to be?"

She gave that some thought. "I want to be kind and loving. I want to be the mom who teaches her kids how to do things. My husband and I argue a lot about how to raise them, so I'd like to be on the same page with him. I'd guess I'd really like to have a more coherent parenting style," she finished.

"How can you learn how to do that?"

"Now, that's a good question!"

After talking it over, Ruth and her husband decided to take parenting classes together, but to go out to dinner beforehand so they could have more relaxed down time with each other. She never totally resolved her mother-lawyer conflict, but she did learn to set clear boundaries for herself about family time. She and her husband worked out what they expected from their kids and began practicing connection and belonging with them.

They were all tiny steps, but they helped her keep her promises to her family and herself and eased her stress when she could not take her children's non-emergency calls at the office.

She scheduled one-on-one time with each child every week, letting them decide what they would do together. That gave her an intentional, nourishing answer to "what's the upside of being home?" It was another tiny step, but it corrected the lopsidedness of her life and relieved her guilt, especially when she recognized that her imbalance resulted from not having equal skill sets for both her family and career poles.

Once she educated herself about parenting, both poles were on equal footing.

Polarity problems are seldom resolved by quitting one thing or the other. Each aspect, Yin and Yang, must be managed because one side is not better than the other. Rather, we need to intentionally grab the positive side of the neglected pole. This way, Ruth was able to hold onto her integrity and not allow one aspect of her life to consume the other.

29 CONTROL WHAT WE CAN

I was with my mother when her physician told her she was headed for Type 2 diabetes.

"He doesn't know anything," she reported to me later, angrily. "I ate a cookie before I had the bloodwork done. That's why the results are off."

At the time, my mother was fifty-five years old, 100 pounds overweight, and only moved when absolutely necessary. She binged on every kind of junk food and suffered diabetes' many complications for the next two decades. When she died at seventy-two, she was on nineteen prescription medications.

You may ask, "Why didn't those medications help?"

The unvarnished answer: prescription medications cannot magically correct lifestyle-induced health issues.

My mother, like so many other people, had built her own bed of ills and then gotten angry and resistant when her physician explained the consequences of not exercising or changing her diet. But in a typical twenty-minute health-care appointment, that was all he could do: anger her. He did not know how to help her overcome her denial, impact her daily decision-making, or change the culture she lived in. Those were all adaptive issues, not technical ones, and adaptive problems cannot be resolved by a top-down edict or prescription.

Healthcare providers are schooled in addressing technical health problems; they diagnose symptoms and provide "do this to relieve that" advice. My mother's physician could cure her pneumonia, for example, because that is a technical problem: a microbe destroyed by a drug. But he did not have the expertise to cure her obesity, because that was an adaptive problem—she caused it, so she had to be involved in solving it.

And that would be no easy feat.

First, she would have had to own the truth of how she got so heavy. Second, she had to decide to stop causing her obesity. And third, she needed to change her ingrained life habits to resolve her weight problem.

That would have meant changing every habit from the moment she woke up to the moment she went to bed—not just her eating habits, but her stress reactions, her self-talk, her self-image, her priorities, and her thought processes. No physician could have possibly fixed that with a simple diet, exercise plan, or prescription drug.

Still, she kept asking for a pill, diet, patch, or false-hope quick-fix for her complex, adaptive problems. There are none. According to the World Health Organization, the four behaviors responsible for most early death in adults in the twenty-first century are (in order, for wealthy nations):

1. Tobacco use
2. Physical inactivity
3. Overweight/Obesity
4. Alcohol abuse

And the numbers are staggering: Almost fifty percent of Americans are obese and suffer from at least one chronic illness. More people do not exercise than do. Nearly twenty percent still smoke, exposing themselves—and those around them—to a known carcinogen.

Yet all those problems are entirely preventable and curable. When we make wellness a priority, our bodies become inhospitable to such adaptive chronic illness as Type 2 diabetes, heart disease, or the thirteen kinds of lifestyle-induced cancer.

Illness Happens

Not all illness is self-generated, of course. Many people unavoidably suffer from technical, not adaptive, chronic diseases and illnesses. My nephew was infected with HIV as a baby. Another family member died at fifty-two from lymphoma—and no amount of life changes could have stopped it. My cousin's breast cancer metastasized to her bones in her forties. A friend became quadriplegic at sixteen from a diving accident. Even my mother's congestive heart failure was the result of childhood Rheumatic fever, which she caught during an epidemic.

Why must some people face the end of their lives in the middle of their lives through no fault of their own or recognizable cause? It remains one of the great mysteries of life.

Our Medical Model's Limitations

When early Greek anatomists dissected the first human body, religious leaders were afraid the cadaver's spirit would wreak havoc on the community, so the anatomists had to cover the entire body except for the part being dissected.

That medical model is still in place today, even though it was established over *2,000 years* ago! Modern health care still mostly focuses on each body part without considering either the body as a whole—or the mind's connection to it. Payment schemes are based on all the ways the body, mind and spirit are broken, each with its own diagnosis and billing code. While there are pockets of innovative thinking in health care, it remains a siloed, sclerotic, and ossified patchwork that is over-focused on treating disease once it has taken hold. Successful corporations may have recognized the need to break out of silo thinking, but modern health care is still hyper-specialized. I know one surgeon who only treats thumbs!

Control What We Can

So, when my mother told her physician, "You don't understand," she was right.

He did not understand what triggered her overeating. He did not understand why she was in denial about her bloodwork. He did not understand her resistance. He did not understand how to heal a patient who did not want to heal herself or was too set in her ways or afraid to consider change. He did not understand how to help her identify an important personal motivator. He could only recommend she "eat less" of the Standard American Diet.

All he could offer, at best, was a Band-Aid for her complex, system-wide health problems. He was the product of his education and he had technical tools to administer. As a physician, he simply did not have the knowledge, training, or perspective to do anything else.

Our antiquated medical model can be lifesaving when faced with a technical problem, such as a broken bone or a burst appendix. But as we saw in a global infectious-virus outbreak, it misses the mark with most of today's adaptive-problems. For those cases, we need to consider potential remedies offered by the big picture, the system-wide versus symptom-level perspective.

You and I are the operators of our own systems. We are the ones who must "heal ourselves." Only we can make the changes to live a long healthy life—no one can do it for us.

That is why I urge you, with all my being and my heart, to choose wellness.

Early Praise for
Choosing Wellness

Choosing Wellness masterfully captures the vulnerability and determination of intentionally changing one's life in big and small ways. O'Grady's riveting life stories reach the very heart of enabling and empowering change in others. She captures the universality of human nature and her personal insights have great meaning for everyone. It is truly a life-changing book!

Jean Johnson PhD, RN, FAAN
Emerita Dean and Professor, School of Nursing,
George Washington University

O'Grady's unvarnished tale of trauma, anger, doubt and ultimate triumph shows us how she walked and self-talked her way out of sabotaging her life in a way that is neither condescending nor preachy. If self-doubt—with or without past trauma—is standing in the way of your health, pick up this beautifully written book. It's profoundly sad in places, but so breezily written that you will not be able to put it down. You will be healthier in both body and mind because of it.

Jayne O'Donnell
USA TODAY Health Policy Reporter;
CEO, Urban Health Media Project

Eileen O'Grady is a survivor—the resilient and gritty kind. Choosing Wellness is filled with wisdom that can only come from experience... her narratives are short, pithy, and brave as she creates windows into our own lives. Reading this is like a deep conversation with a caring friend. She reminds us that at every turn, we get to choose to live our lives fully and bravely.

Gregory Pawlson MD, MPH
Faculty and Coach National Geriatrics
Palliative Care Fellows Program

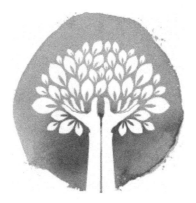